||| | | ||||||||||||||| ||| ||| |||
I0132384

Hello Chiropractic,
Goodbye Colic

Copyright © 2010
Steven L. Kooyers, D.C.

ALL RIGHTS RESERVED

FOR INFORMATION CONTACT:
Steven L. Kooyers, D.C.
780 B. N. State St.
Ukiah, Ca 95482
Email: stevekooyers@yahoo.com

THANK YOU

I would like to thank some special people for helping me. To Jo, I am especially thankful. She has been so patient with me.

Jill Hannum is my longtime friend. She is also my tireless editor who turned my rambling verbiage into concise thoughts. Without her exceptional input, this book would never have made it. I appreciate you, Jill.

I would also like to thank my teachers at Palmer College of Chiropractic in Davenport, Iowa. Their high ethics and principled instruction forged a lifelong purpose in me. They showed me the value of specificity and taught me that one specific vertebral adjustment beats a thousand "manipulations."

Lastly, I would like to thank my many patients who exhibited such gracious patience when they entered my office while I busily typed away. Now I can say it, folks: thanks, and *it's finally done!*

I dedicate this book to all young parents.
I hope that it helps you
to make informed choices.
May it give you blissful babies.

TABLE OF CONTENTS

PREFACE   6

1: THE KEY PLAYERS: COLIC,
    SUBLUXATION, CHIROPRACTIC   18

2: WHAT CAUSES COLIC?   28

3: SUBLUXATION AND THE
    NEUROANATOMY OF THE NEWBORN   48

4: FINDING A BABY-FRIENDLY
    CHIROPRACTOR   66

5: YOUR BABY'S FIRST VISIT
    TO THE CHIROPRACTOR   82

6: WHAT TO EXPECT AFTER THE
    ADJUSTMENT— FOLLOW UP VISITS,
    AVOIDING "RELAPSE"   90

7: WHAT IF CHIROPRACTIC
    DOESN'T HELP?   96

8: BREAST-FEEDING---A GREAT COLIC
    PREVENTATIVE   106

9: MEDICINE RESISTS CHANGE   112

ABOUT THE AUTHOR   131

GLOSSARY OF TERMS   135

PREFACE

Perhaps I was predisposed from a very early age to believe not only in the efficacy of chiropractic but also in its power to vanquish colic. My mother often told the story of the "miracle cure" of my older brother's colic. In the late spring of 1944, my mother and infant brother were on a train somewhere in Idaho, and my brother had been crying for hours. Finally, as my mom tells it, "A stranger got up and walked over to me. He said, 'Ma'am, would you mind if I help your baby?' I said, 'No, please do!' Well, he just put his hand on little Ronny's head, and he held it there for a minute. Ronny stopped crying right then and there. That stranger went to another car and rode the rest of the trip there. Ron's colic never did come back."

I'll bet that the stranger was either an osteopath or a chiropractor trained in cranial correction. Back then, both professions were scorned for their alternative techniques. It's very likely this man felt compelled to help a crying infant, yet wanted no recognition—many such practitioners went to jail in those days for "practicing medicine" without a license. I'm sure he knew he could help Ron, and I'm sure he was desperate for some peace and quiet, so he took the risk of approaching my mother.

Chiropractors no longer go to jail for helping babies with colic, but we still suffer from the fallout of decades of virulent anti-chiropractic propaganda by the American Medical Association and other organizations of allopaths. (I discuss this at length in Chapter 8.) No parent fears taking a baby to a pediatrician, but calming very nervous mothers is often the first "adjustment" of her first visit to a chiropractor. Here is a quite typical scenario:

A FIRST VISIT

Angie, a very young mother, had never been to a chiropractor before, and she didn't know me at all. I could sense her anxiety as she handed me her beautiful baby girl. I had seen such tired, desperate young mothers many times before, and I felt I knew her story already. I could only think of one thing to say: "Don't worry; I won't harm your baby." Tears of relief welled up in her eyes and she gave a nervous, thin little laugh. If it hadn't been for baby Monique's constant crying and writhing, Angie would never have entrusted her precious new daughter to a strange doctor with a strange treatment method.

On examination, I found two subluxations in Monique's spine—one was high in the neck and the other low in the back. Her spine was the stiffest I had seen in years, and she cried even louder as I gently touched each sore spot. About two minutes after I adjusted her spine, Monique stopped crying. In five minutes, she was fast asleep with a look of utter relief on her face. Angie couldn't get over it and kept saying, "If I hadn't seen it, I wouldn't believe it!"

Within a week, Monique was sleeping through the nights and so were her parents. Her colic was practically gone. She went from six hours of crying per day to twenty minutes. I told Angie, "If she reacts like other babies have, by next week the colic will be totally gone. After that, she'll only cry when she needs to; when she's wet, hungry or frightened—just like any healthy baby."

One week later, Angie brought a peacefully sleeping Monique to my office, and she filled me in about the birth trauma, the medical run-around and the ineffective medical treatments the baby had endured. After 30 years of practice, I thought that I had heard it all, but there was a new element to Angie's story that made me especially angry. The doctors had diagnosed Monique's problem as "acid reflux" and prescribed Zantac! My anger extended from the individual MD to the whole medical system that could treat an infant so abusively, and that anger motivated me to write this book. I want others to learn the truth about colic, so that as many babies as possible can be spared having to endure this painful condition.

Angie also told me of the arguments she'd had with her parents, her in-laws and her doctors before visiting my office. Her father had said that he would disown her if she took the baby to a chiropractor. Her husband was so burned out from the constant crying that he just didn't care any more. Her pediatrician told her that chiropractic was "dangerous" for babies and announced that if she followed through on her plan, she'd have to find a new pediatrician. As she poured her heart out about the hurdles she had had to overcome, my heart went out to Angie and to all the other parents who have to make tough choices in order to help their babies.

THE PHILOSOPHY BEHIND MY PRACTICE

I believe that each of us has within a tiny spark of the intelligent force that drives the universe. Call it the Creator or any of its many other names that are used all across the world. The discoverer of chiropractic, Daniel D. Palmer, called it the "Innate Intelligence", a capacity or power deep inside your body that maintains the healthy expression of your life force.

Like Palmer, I believe that we were created to be healthy and that good health is not luck or an accident. When we are not healthy, there's a reason for it; and by adjusting subluxations, we are removing blockages in order to free up the power of Innate Intelligence. Once unblocked, it can again send healthy messages that make it possible for you to regain that vital but delicate balance of energy deep inside your body that is crucial to optimum health.

I honor the body's Innate Intelligence and believe strongly that people who are not healthy should try the safe, low-tech methods of regaining their health before turning to the often risky, high-tech approaches. If I were to set up a national healthcare plan, I'd turn the common patterns on their head: a thorough chiropractic evaluation would precede the prescription for drugs and/or surgery (barring, of course, traumatic emergencies); massage and emotional support—perhaps a thousand hugs—would precede antidepressants or electroshock therapy; acupuncture would precede the administration of dangerous weight loss chemicals that damage the heart or "stomach stapling" surgery. I'd commission medical schools to promote a balanced (not merely a chemical) look at the body and would urge them to stop treating symptoms and start treating people. I would advocate a paradigm shift in medical curriculae all across America that would continue to train some doctors to save lives but would also train some doctors to change lives. Both are admirable goals and both are sorely needed—though I wonder if, on reflection, it isn't best to change lives first, then see whether more drastic, technological intervention is still needed.

Unfortunately, most Americans are in awe of modern technology. They equate it with health care, think that a doctor is almost a god, and in general are sure that if one pill doesn't cure them, more pills will. That's a lot of ingrained, wrongful thinking about healthcare.

Society's thinking is growing increasingly medicalized every day. Drug companies pay for medical schools, so the medical students learn only drugs and surgery. Today, pharmaceutical companies (Big Phama) buy huge amounts of television time and lobby our government extremely heavily. When our society sees only drugs as the path to health, we will have lost a great deal of wisdom from the past. When we train doctors to see only drugs as the path to health, we have lost the present. And when we needlessly drug our children, we will lose our future.

In my philosophy, true health comes from the amazing life force deep inside your body that controls and coordinates millions of your actions every single day of your life and charges you with energy and purpose. There are many ways that your Innate Intelligence can be impaired, and spinal subluxation is not only one of these ways, it is the single most overlooked way—because nobody looks for it except chiropractors.

When I detect subluxation in a baby, I feel compassion for the parents because they also feel their baby's pain, but I also feel confidence and hope because I know that once the baby has been adjusted, good things will start happening. Innate Intelligence wants a happy, healthy baby! I also know that I'm not doing the healing, I simply get to play a part by removing the obstacle to healing. That is a wonderful thing to do for a baby. Very few people can do that, and when you think about it, it's really pretty cool—we chiropractors touch people, and then they get better. I like that.

I am honored to be able to witness awesome recoveries and to be a part of something so ... universal. It is truly humbling and truly gratifying.

THE MANDATORY DISCLAIMERS

Our society is chock-full of lawyers and people ready to use them. Sometimes, we really need a lawyer and a good healthy lawsuit—without the legal process, we chiropractors would never have won our landmark antitrust and restraint of trade suit against the American Medical Association (Wilk et al, v. AMA et al, 1977). That said, I need to set forth the following disclaimers:

Chiropractic is not a substitute for an MD's care. There are potentially serious medical problems that need to be ruled out before you bring your infant to a chiropractor. Pre-screening your infant to rule out dangerous pre-existing conditions and making the diagnosis of colic are the role of your pediatrician. (It is likely one reason chiropractors get such awesome results with colic; the dangerous and difficult cases have been pre-screened.)

Chiropractic doesn't "cure" anything. Technically, a "cure" is something like giving antivenin for snakebite; it is a specific remedy to alleviate a specific symptom. In chiropractic school, we are taught not to "chase symptoms" but to balance the body; which, in turn will

14

address the symptoms. Indeed, in many states, it is not legal for a chiropractor to even to talk about "cure"—it can lead to a law suit for practicing medicine without a license. Early chiropractic textbooks, circa 1900, referred to cures, but that was a time when every healthcare faction was obsessed with "the cure" for all disease and infirmity. Osteopathy, allopathy, naturopathy, homeopathy, chiropractic, naprapathy, the Ralstonites, the Kelloggs— all claimed to have "the cure" for all disease. Today, when we hear "cure" we think of some external agent (think antivenin again), and most cures remain in the domain of allopathy. In chiropractic, we are not in the curing business. If you see the "C word" in this book, understand that I have used it in the generic sense of the word. Chiropractic doesn't actually cure colic even though it certainly looks like a cure when it's successful. Technically speaking, chiropractic cures nothing.

Results vary. Many factors affect outcomes, and a chiropractor can address only a few of them. The parent has a role in the healing process as well, and even if all parties do everything right, there's still a chance the colic will persist. Studies show that chiropractic is successful in over 92% of colic cases, but sometimes it will fail.

Chiropractors vary. Among chiropractors there is a wide variation in adjusting skills, opinions and philosophies. This might be due to the fact that chiropractic education is not as rigidly formatted as that of medical schools. This allows individual practitioners considerable creative freedom, which can spawn excellent chiropractors but is not always a good thing. Chiropractic is "operator dependent", and the public lacks guidelines to determine who's good and who's not. I always advise that if you don't get what you want from one chiropractor, try another.

Corroborating data. Although I have quoted studies and statistics from a wide array of websites, I have not personally verified their accuracy. The sites are listed at the back of this book, and they're just a click away if you want to delve more deeply into any of them This book is intended to be used primarily as a primer to get parents to start thinking about chiropractic and colic. It is decidedly not a textbook—I'm a hands-on kind of person who would rather fix a problem than read studies and statistics about it. Which is why I must stress the following:

This book reflects my own personal opinions, not those of any organizations, institutions or colleges. While some of my opinions dovetail with conventional chiropractic training, others don't. If my opinions matched everyone else's, I wouldn't have written this book.

CHAPTER 1

INTRODUCING THE KEY PLAYERS:
COLIC, SUBLUXATION, CHIROPRACTIC

WHAT IS COLIC?

The medical dictionary defines colic as: "A symptom complex seen in infants under three months of age, characterized by paroxysmal abdominal pain and frantic crying." A diagnosis of "colic" is made when a baby cries for three or more hours per day, for three or more days per week, for three or more weeks. This is called the "law of threes". That's a lot of crying. If you scan the Internet sites on colic, you'll read that the cause of colic is "unknown", that it's harmless, that one in five babies gets it. You'll see it referred to as "normal", as "gas", as a problem that will eventually go away. The world of allopathic medicine, as I will stress throughout this book, admits to not knowing the cause of colic and none of the treatments it offers works very well. Like most chiropractors, I know the cause of colic, and because I know the cause, I can fix almost every case. Here is the core of this book in a nutshell: The cause of colic is spinal subluxation. Chiropractic care corrects spinal subluxation, and in response colic disappears.

SUBLUXATION—THE BASIC PROBLEM DEFINED

In a normal, healthy spine, each vertebra is supposed to participate in concert with each of its neighbors—each vertebra moves a little in just the right way so that all of them can move together in painless flexibility. This is "normal alignment" and when you have it, you have a healthy body. A subluxation is, at first, a disturbance of that normal, healthy relationship between adjacent vertebrae. Subluxated vertebrae don't play their part in normal movement and load sharing patterns—they become either very stiff or much too mobile. This is referred to as "altered motoricity of paired vertebrae", and it is one of the hallmarks of subluxation both in infants and adults.

Given sufficient reinforcement, the subluxation affects the spinal nerve roots. This can lead to target organ malfunction. (Each of the 64 nerve roots supplies specific organs, these are the "targets" for those nerves.) Given more time and/or severity, this can lead to illness, the exact nature and level of which depends upon the location of the subluxation and the patient's resistance, lifestyle, genetics, etc.

WHAT IS CHIROPRACTIC?

Chiropractic is a drugless healthcare system that works with the body's inherent recuperative powers. It was first advocated by Daniel David Palmer in 1895. History shows attempts at spinal care dating back to before the ancient Egyptians, but these references were only for alleviating back pain. DD, as Palmer was known, was the first to advocate that the nerve system played a dominant role in health and illness. He proposed the chiropractic "adjustment" as a means to impact the nerve system positively, with the intent of restoring homeostasis or optimum function of all the body's vital parts. Not long after giving his first few "treatments", DD advocated wellness-based care via maintenance spinal alignments. Thus, he was the very first practitioner of any discipline to advocate prevention-based healthcare.

In today's modern healthcare world, this is still an advanced idea; but imagine how radically advanced it was in 1895 for DD Palmer to postulate that the relationship between the body's structure and its healthy functioning has a pivotal role in restoring and preserving optimal health.

A chiropractor or DC (Doctor of Chiropractic) uses natural methods as his or her tools. These include nutrition, supplementation, exercise, hygienic measures (fresh air, exercise, positive thinking, etc.), and, of course, the chiropractic adjustment. The adjustment is performed upon subluxated vertebrae, with the express purpose of correcting nerve interference, and the term refers to a process that includes the procedure preparatory to the chiropractic thrust, the thrust itself and the post-check. In order to adjust a vertebra properly, chiropractors always go through a short protocol. First, of course, we determine whether there is a subluxation. If so, we decide the "Line of Correction"—the direction of thrust. For example, I might decide that what's called for is a line that could be described as "straight lateral to medial with just a bit of torque." Next, we assess the depth of thrust, amount of recoil, tissue pull, stabilization and traction. Then we "pre-load the articulation" (i.e., correctly position the point of contact) and prepare to administer the thrust. After we pre-set these perameters, we perform the adjustment.

Adjustments are made with one intent—to correct subluxations in order to achieve full and uncompromised nerve system communication. That is, to help the body achieve a state where its innate recuperative power is flowing at one hundred percent. This is the baseline for optimal health, and that's what chiropractic shoots for— optimal health.

Chiropractors see subluxation as an illness vector that is overlooked by almost all other health care professions. In some cases, this single vector can be the difference between health and illness. In most cases, subluxation plays a less dominant role. Chiropractors work to clear out subluxation, regardless of its apparent role in any current health picture.

To that aim, chiropractors treat millions of healthy people who have no symptoms at all. Our treatment isn't based upon symptoms or illness, although symptoms or illness are what bring people to our offices for treatment. This is the source of much misunderstanding and confusion, especially from allopathically oriented people who are trained to equate symptoms with illness and lack of symptoms with health.

Chiropractic is a natural method. It has its limits, and all good chiropractors respect them. When we see cases that exceed these limits, we refer them to other health professionals for appropriate care.

HOW DO NEWBORNS BECOME SUBLUXATED?

The answer to this question can be found in the perils of the journey from womb to delivery room and beyond. Imagine yourself as a fetus...

Your first few months inside the womb are blissful. There's unlimited space, and you float freely. Gradually, things start getting cramped. You scrunch into a curve, trying to find enough room. Your head and body keep growing ... the room is shrinking!

You kick, to try to get more room; you try a few blows with those tiny arms. Nothing works! You keep growing and soon the womb begins to squeeze back! Contractions start and the uterine walls squeeze your head and neck against the pelvic bones. During labor the uterus is the strongest muscle in the mother's body. Using your whole body for leverage, the uterus rams your head and neck into and through the birth canal.

As soon as your head exits the canal, hands grasp it with a twisting, pulling motion. You have no muscle tone to defend against such traction. As the doctor twists your head to one side, delicate, undeveloped muscles and tissues get wrenched—you've never before made a movement you didn't initiate! If you feel pain, you can't express it since you don't yet have any air in your lungs.

As your body finally slides out, hands grab you by the legs, swat you on the butt, and dangle you in the cold air. Then someone sticks a tube in your mouth, weighs you, dangles you, and stabs you with needles, wraps you in a scratchy blanket. Now gravity takes over, robbing you of your previous mobility. Your head weighs so much that you cannot even move it.

Though most modern births aren't necessarily so traumatic being born can still be a very tough event. Some babies will become subluxated during or shortly after the birth process. Others will become subluxated in the first few days post partum, either at the hands of the hospital staff or the family. Babies can also become subluxated via another source—pain. There are many sources of pain in a birth room, from the first pinprick all the way to circumcision. A baby's nervous system is not developed enough to route pain properly. Intense or unexpected pain for a neonate can result in subluxation, which (especially in infants) is more a neural event than an osteological event. (For a detailed explanation of this phenomenon, see Chapter 3.)

It's common to hear someone dismiss the idea of subluxation—not only that it might occur, but that it might cause a real problem if it does occur. People say, "Oh, my neck goes out, but it doesn't bother me, so it couldn't hurt a baby." Babies are not little adults, and this is the kind of reasoning that also allows adults to expose them to punk rock concerts and Monster Truck rallies. Babies' ears are not like adult ears. A baby's ear canal is comparatively short and wide, allowing sounds to penetrate that will easily damage a baby's hearing but will leave the adult's hearing more or less intact. A baby's eyes are more susceptible to light, a baby's membranes are more susceptible to heat (even a too-warm bottle) and cold.

I emphasize that infants are not miniature adults. Subluxated adults rarely display the severity of symptoms that occur in pediatric subluxation. Atlas subluxation in an adult might only cause migraines or sinus problems; in a newborn baby, it can result in failure to thrive, colic, cardiac arrhythmia and other serious internal problems.

FROM MY FILES—OCTOBER 1979:

Elaine had been crying non-stop since she'd been born seven days earlier. She had been born at home and was a totally organic baby, but she had more muscle tension than any baby I've ever touched! I found a high thoracic subluxation, at T3.

When I adjusted T3, she quit crying just long enough to give me a really dirty look, then took a breath and began crying again. But this time, it was in a much different cadence and tone. It sounded for the world like she was cursing at me! After five minutes, she stopped crying. When I saw her again the next day, she was cooing. Elaine required just the one adjustment; her colic never returned.

CHAPTER 2
WHAT CAUSES COLIC?

COMMON MYTHS ABOUT COLIC

Practically everything you've been told about colic is untrue; that's one of my core messages.

Once your pediatrician has ruled out other possible causes for your baby's constant crying and has diagnosed colic, it's almost as if he or she goes on automatic pilot. Naming colic is not the same as curing it, but sometimes doctors seem to think that putting a label on it will make the parents sleep better. What follows is a look at the common myths about colic. If you have a baby with colic, you will have heard almost all of them.

1. The Cause Of Colic Is Unknown. Medically speaking, this is true. In medical parlance, the term for a disease of unknown origin is "idiopathic." But whatever the moniker, it's important to remember that in spite of efforts to treat colic for centuries, the cause still eludes medical experts.

Scrutinize the literature, read the websites, or ask most doctors and you may encounter the word "idiopathic" and descriptions of symptoms, and discussion of treatment, but no investigation of cause. I have a problem with that. How can one fix something without knowing its cause? I would suggest that perhaps this is why medicine has limited success with colic. The cause of colic is <u>not</u> unknown: it is subluxation.

2. It's Harmless. <u>Never</u> let a doctor tell you that colic is harmless. Just imagine how your own body would feel after hours of high volume screaming and all-out crying. This kind of whole-body involvement has a wide range of possible effects, none of them good. In addition, a constantly screaming baby is treated very differently than a quiet baby, and it is most probable that he/she knows that. People avoid a baby with colic; positive feedback via eye contact and smiles just doesn't happen; and a lot of important developmental feedback just isn't happening. At the most dangerous end of this spectrum, the constant crying can drive adults and siblings to distraction and suddenly they're shaking the baby to try to silence it. "Shaken Baby Syndrome" kills. An infant has no muscle tone to protect its delicate spinal column, and it only takes

a split second of shaking to be fatal because shaking whiplashes the head and neck, causing tearing of the delicate upper spinal cord tissue. Colic is not harmless.

3. It's An Immature Digestive Tract. This myth is just plain ... dumb. Yet some otherwise bright doctors parrot it, ignoring lessons learned in first-year embryology. There is no such thing as an immature digestive tract in a mature baby. A full-term baby is not a cake, which can be overdone on the outside and still gooey on the inside. The digestive tract develops right along with the other organs and systems of the body, it doesn't lag behind them.

The many Internet websites devoted to colic make no special mention of premature babies. Yet if an immature digestive tract really caused colic, "preemies" would be front-page news on those sites. Premature babies really do have immature organs, but they don't have an increased incidence of colic. Conversely, over-term babies, whose GI tracts are theoretically more mature, ought to be immune to colic—but they are not. Obviously, intestinal tract immaturity is not a cause of colic.

4. It's Gas. Gas does not cause colic any more than fruit flies cause grapes to rot. Yes, plenty of colicky babies have gas. But so do plenty of babies who don't get colic. So how can gas be the cause? Ask any mother of a colicky baby about gas—long after the baby burps or farts, the crying continues. If gas caused the crying, it should stop, at least briefly, when the gas is expelled.

Now, gas certainly is associated with colic. Often, when a baby is in pain, gas can be created because the pain inhibits gastric motility and disturbs digestion (see Chapter 3). But gas does not cause colic. I've adjusted many infants and their crying often stops immediately; even when they still have a big, tight belly full of gas.

If MDs really believed that gas bubbles cause colic, wouldn't they prescribe something to stop the gas, and wouldn't that work? If it were that simple, an antacid would cure colic.

THE MARITAL IMPACTS OF COLIC:
A Fact-based Scenario

John, 32, and Mary, 31 have a 5-week old baby girl, Alice. Jason, 13, is John's son by a previous marriage. Alice has been crying constantly since birth. John works two jobs. Mary had a job, until she got pregnant. Alice's expensive medical tests came back 'normal'. The doctor said; "Alice has colic. It's harmless; she'll outgrow it." The family tried to sleep through the constant crying, but couldn't. John and Mary tried rocking her and walking the floor with her. Because she didn't cry as much in a moving car, they took shifts driving Alice around all night. John started being late for work and was fired him from one job. John is obsessed with money woes—medical bills, alimony, a hospital lien on his property. His son is starting to get distant and his father tells him that a real man takes better care of his family.

The crying and the stress have practically dried up Mary's breast milk, she's barely slept since the delivery and now has postpartum depression. John grows more distant each day. Mary, too, is worried about the medical bills. She might get a job, but the daycare centers say no colicky babies are allowed! Mary felt more and more trapped, there seemed to be no way out...

Jason needs attention from his parents, gets none and the constant screaming gets on his nerves! His grades drop; he starts staying out late. A few more sleepless nights and somebody just might shake Baby Alice. Divorce seems likely. Nobody can get any sleep. And all because of one tiny, screaming baby!

5. Colic Helps Develop Lung Power. Some doctors claim that colic is nature's way of developing lung strength. If constant screaming is necessary to develop lungs, why don't all babies do it? If it's truly needed, we should see analogous behavior in other mammals. Baby primates don't cry constantly, neither do most human babies. In fact, colic doesn't usually manifest in all the kids in a family; not all children who share the same genetics for lung development, get colic. The lungpower argument does not fit the laws of biology.

6. It's Normal. I am baffled that the medical profession tries to pull this wool over our eyes. You have a baby that cries and screams constantly. What is normal about that? How can a healthcare professional expect you to believe that?

When a condition is "Normal," most people do it, feel it or get it. Normal means "harmless", "ordinary" and "common." Normal means that things are ok. There is nothing normal about colic.

7. Your Baby Will Grow Out of It. Yes, eventually all babies "grow out of" their colic. The oldest child I ever saw

with colic was 15 months old. But pediatricians are classically optimistic in their predictions to mothers. One of my infant patient's mothers told me that her pediatrician at first told her, "Your baby will grow out of in a few months." When that didn't happen, the doctor threw up his hands and said the baby would grow out of it "in a couple of years!" Why wait that long? Would you accept this response for any other childhood problem—scoliosis, bowed legs, crossed eyes?

8. You Got One Of The Colicky Ones. This is a variation of the "It's normal" myth. The implication is that you won some kind of "bad kid lottery". The doctor expects you to believe that somehow, although most kids never get colic, you won the lottery; you got one that did, and you should just put up with it. A doctor who says this just wants you to hush up and take it lying down.

If your baby had been born with a tail, you wouldn't just accept that you'd been dealt a bad hand of cards. To me, colic is almost as abnormal as a tail. It's not normal and you didn't just get a "cranky one". If you went to a kennel, picked out a puppy, and on arriving home discovered that you picked out a loser, it might be fair to say; "Oh, you picked the worst pup from that litter ... too bad." But having a baby is not the same thing, and there is no such thing as the "bad baby lottery"!

Here is the bottom line: Believing in myths won't help your baby.

FROM MY FILES—JANUARY 2005:

Madelyn came to me at 13 months. She had averaged four hours of screaming per day since she was two weeks old. Her pediatricians had promised she'd "outgrow it in a few months." When I first saw her, she was absolutely screaming. It was the most urgent cry for help I've ever heard. I just HAD to help that little girl.

Before even filling out any paperwork, I reached into the car seat and palpated her cranial bones, which desperately needed correction. I timed my corrective movements so that every time she inhaled, I gently nudged the occiput. In five minutes, she went to sleep.

While a flabbergasted Laurie filled out the paperwork, she kept looking at Madelyn as if the baby were a Martian. Finally, she exclaimed; "That's the first time she's ever shut up!" Madelyn had never slept for more than half an hour or so before she'd wake up screaming. After her first treatment, she slept for five hours straight.

Madelyn needed three more treatments over two weeks. She had been a suction-cup delivery, with the cup applied to her head in order to pull her out of the birth canal. I presume that the suction force caused her subluxation, as her patterns were rare for naturally delivered babies. (Atlas subluxation, occiput fault. Four treatments, fifteen days. Zero colic after second week)

FOOLISH TREATMENTS

Giving Drugs for Colic. In spite of not knowing what causes colic, doctors have begun prescribing drugs for colicky babies. A mother who brought her baby to me in May 2007 had recently had her pediatrician prescribe drugs for "acid reflux". This baffles me. Infants don't have a well developed "swallow and hold it down" reflex. They normally spit up until the coordinated peristaltic reflex develops. This is a normal, developmental process that every baby must learn. Until then, there will be normal regurgitation. It's not a disease, it's not "acid reflux", and it does not need prescription drugs!

Resorting to such a prescription ignores normal developmental physiology. Imagine if the doctor prescribed Ritalin because the newborn couldn't speak yet! A baby doesn't need drugs to learn to speak, it's a learned act—just like swallowing. Drugs won't help a baby learn to swallow.

Treatments and Remedies You Find Online. On the Internet you'll see herbal remedies, Homeopathic and Naturopathic remedies, herbs, Lullabands, hot baths,

Tucker wedges and home remedies—all touted as "cures" for colic. (You'll also see some valuable counseling on breast-feeding, changing formulas, maternal nutrition, etc, and I'll discuss a few of these later, as they may make sense for the 8-9% of babies with colic that do not respond to chiropractic adjustment.) In a random scan of ten websites on colic, I found recommendations for 40 different treatments! To my thinking, when you see this many treatments for one problem, you can be assured that none of them really works very well!

THE *REAL* CAUSE OF COLIC

Like most chiropractors, I know the cause of colic. Chiropractors achieve results in over 92% of all colic cases, with an average of 3.8 visits, in only two weeks. (This statistic is an average of the findings of three separate studies—Wilberg, et al., Klougart, et al., and Nilsson.[1]) If I can fix almost every case with just a few

---

[1] A study in the *Journal of Manipulative and Physiologic Therapeutics* (Wiberg JMM, Nordsteen J, Nilsson N. "The Short-Term Effect of Spinal Manipulation in the Treatment of Infantile Colic: A Randomized Controlled Clinical Trial with a Blinded Observer". *J Manipulative Physiol Ther* 1999 (Oct); 22 (8): 517-522) concluded, "Spinal manipulation is effective in relieving infantile colic". For a period of two weeks, half of the subjects underwent chiropractic spinal

treatments, I must know the cause. As I've said, it's spinal subluxation.

That sounds almost too simple, even to me. You're probably thinking; "If that's all it is, why didn't my real doctor find it?" Not only are MDs predisposed to discount DCs and chiropractic in general (see "Why Didn't My Doctor Recommend a Chiropractor?" in Chapter 8), but your doctor has no training in detecting spinal subluxation—not even a single hour in medical school. You can't expect the medical establishment to find

---

manipulation, while the other half received the drug dimethicone. All of the adjusted babies stayed in the study, while only 64% of the dimethicone babies completed the two-week study. In the course of the study, the children being adjusted saw a 67% reduction in crying and the drug therapy group saw only a 38% reduction in crying. The mean number of adjustments given during the two-week study was 3.8.

The findings of this report resemble the results of "The efficacy of chiropractic spinal adjustments as a treatment protocol in the management of infantile colic" by Mercer and Cook of South Africa. Similarly, in a study of 316 children a satisfactory result occurred within two weeks in 94% of the cases receiving chiropractic care. (Klougart N, Nilsson N, Jacobsen J. "Infantile colic Treated by Chiropractors: A Prospective Study of 316 Cases". *J Manipulative Physiol Ther* 1989 (Aug); 12 (4): 281-8.) In yet another study of 132 infants with colic, 91% of the parents reported an improvement occurring after an average of two to three manipulations. (Nilsson N. "Infant Colic and Chiropractic". *Eur J Chiropr* 1985; 33 (4): 264-265.)

something it doesn't know how to look for, indeed, often doesn't even believe exists!

Chiropractors devote years of training to finding and fixing spinal subluxation. After earning a college degree, chiropractors spend approximately as many hours in chiropractic school as MDs spend in medical school (@ 2200 hours). Like MDs, chiropractors must pass rigorous national and state board examinations before being licensed to practice. Unlike medical students, students of chiropractic focus on the musculoskeletal system (50-60% of the hours vs. less than 1% of the hours) and on how to treat it. After we are licensed, chiropractors must attend twelve hours a year (California DCs) in re-licensing training, of which a minimum of four hours must be on adjusting technique. We are the only doctors with this training, the only experts in subluxation.

HOW SPINAL SUBLUXATION CAUSES COLIC

When an infant has a subluxation anywhere along the spine, it can cause colic (or other problems as well). Here's what is going on: The subluxation can cause pressure on the spinal nerve roots and irritate the brainstem and vagus nerve. This irritation can cause a newborn's digestive system to go haywire in ways that can make the digestive tract <u>seem</u> to be "immature", even though it's not. Painful gas forms because the digestive tract is both malfunctioning and irritated. That's why colic remains even after you change what the baby is eating. It's an internal problem, not an external one. As long as the baby remains subluxated, the baby's gut tract stays irritated, regardless of the type of food in the tract.

Chiropractic care corrects the spinal subluxation that caused the gastrointestinal tract symptoms. The tract then calms down and goes back to digesting food instead of fermenting it. You start seeing a happy baby.

The basic theory that chiropractors operate under when it comes to colic is that it's not the food; it's the subluxation, which impairs normal assimilation, which results in gas and crying. It's not perfect, but for a working theory, it's close enough.

We can test this theory easily; let us adjust the baby until the subluxations go away. That should stop the crying, if our theory is accurate. Given chiropractic's excellent track record with colic cases, our theory must be fairly correct.

As with most clinical procedures, so too with chiropractic adjusting—when we bring pure academic theory into the real world, there is usually a bit of unavoidable slippage. In about one case in ten, we won't be able to help the baby. We are working from the outside of the body on an internal structural dysfunction, which exists underneath several layers of muscle, fat and fascia. Despite this disadvantage, an average success rate of nine out of ten cases relieved within two weeks is proof enough for most of us.

DOING YOUR HOMEWORK

Many conscientious parents, especially those who have no personal experience with chiropractic, will want to do further research on the benefits of chiro-practic for infants (and perhaps for themselves). The first place most people go to find information these days is the web. If you put "colic, chiropractic" into your preferred search engine, you'll get a long list of sites, including www.chiroweb.com, www.holisticonline.com, and www.icpca.org, the site for chiropractic pediatrics. Many of these sites provide thoughtful, balanced information.

Searching the websites on chiropractic, it won't take you long to see that some champion chiropractic care and others are decidedly and vigorously anti-chiropractic. As a lay person, how can you determine which site/poster makes valid claims? I believe that there are two basic reasons for hosting an anti-chiropractic website. The first is ignorance. The second is animosity.

Some of these sites host anti-chiropractic opinions that have actually been posted by someone who is a chiropractor. Like any profession, we have our malcontents. My personal surmise is that a DC who feels compelled to badmouth his own profession might not have learned how to apply the art, science and philosophy of chiropractic as it was intended. For them, chiropractic "didn't work" and rather than augment their training, they go on the attack. I'm sure that sometimes money changes hands—many interests may feel they will benefit from the publication of an anti-chiropractic position, especially when it comes from someone with a DC degree.

I want to stress that the chiropractic profession displays a wide range of talents, both philosophical and technical. When practiced by ethical chiropractors with a solid philosophical base, spinal adjusting is safe and effective. When used by individuals without an ethical, philosophical and artistic base or clinical proficiency, "chiropractic" results will be abysmal.

Some chiropractors may genuinely believe that the training they received confers no benefit on their patients. Others may savor the notoriety they receive from expressing a contrarian opinion. Still others are, I've noted, apparently motivated by the seductive illusion that the medical profession might approve of an anti-chiropractic stance, and thus will approve of someone who expresses it. I see it as being akin to a "Munchausen by Proxy" situation. This is where a parent intentionally harms a child in order to get close to/command the attention of a medical doctor. Thus, the DC "harms the profession" to gain favor with the MD. For example, in 2005 I read a paper by a chiropractor stating that adjusting the Atlas vertebra from the right side would cause a stroke in virtually every case. This came as a surprise to me, as I've adjusted at least fifty thousand atlas vertebrae from the right side, without causing any adverse side effects whatsoever. No credible anatomical, biological or chiropractic reason exists for avoiding right side atlas subluxations. Checking further, I learned that an anti-chiropractic group had purchased the author's opinion.

There are a few chiropractors that make a lucrative living selling anti-chiropractic opinions. Some testify against chiropractic in court cases where damages awarded for soft tissue injuries, in car crashes, for example, are often high. Others become insurance company "hired guns". They are paid well to audit honest chiropractic insurance claims and then systematically deny every single claim. My first personal encounter with such a person was at a technique seminar in 2006. His demonstration "adjustment" on a colleague resembled a criminal assault and left the "patient" in tears for ten minutes. Given his crude technique, the man failed to get results in private practice, his practice failed and he went broke. I ran into him on the street two years later and he bragged, "Steve, I'm making five times what I used to make in practice!" When I appeared disinterested, he continued, "Yeah, man, I'm working as an insurance expert. All I have to do is deny, deny, deny! *It's easy!"* So, when you encounter anti-chiropractic websites, it pays to investigate the source.

You might also encounter another form of prejudice while researching chiropractic and children. This form is deceptive, as it damns with faint praise. It establishes trust by first conceding some benefits to chiropractic, only to conclude with a commonly encountered scare tactic—"Oh, chiropractic; it's good for some things, but don't let them touch your neck!"

Comments like this always demonstrate not only prejudice against chiropractic but also extremely limited knowledge of chiropractic care. Occasionally a patient may, for a variety of reasons, refuse neck treatment—one of my patients associated having her neck touched with a traumatic childhood event, others have post-surgical considerations or other legitimate contraindications. As our first concern is for the patient's welfare and wishes, ethical chiropractors always respect such (rare) requests.

But no such justification exists for the blanket statement "Don't let 'em touch the neck." Spinal subluxation, especially in the neck, can wreak havoc upon the body's health. Asking me not to adjust a subluxation in an adult's or an infant's neck would not only severely limit my effectiveness but would also be asking me to do something unethical. If asked to allow a baby to remain subluxated, I would not touch the neck and I would respectfully decline to treat the baby at all. In chiropractic, we are concerned with two things; the patient's health and our reputation for getting sick people well. By knowingly allowing a subluxation to exist in the cervical spine, I would be jeopardizing both.

To ask us to avoid the neck, based purely upon an outdated but widely circulated prejudice, is a huge disservice to chiropractic patients of any age.

CHAPTER 3

SUBLUXATION AND THE NEUROANATOMY OF THE NEWBORN

AN INFANT'S NERVOUS SYSTEM IS UNIQUELY OPEN TO INPUT

There are some important differences between a baby's nerve system and an adult's. For instance, the baby's brain stem extends well down into the neck, sometimes as far as the third cervical vertebra. As the baby grows and the spinal column elongates, the brain stem gradually retracts into the skull. The brain stem controls all vital functions—heart rate, breathing, digestion, etc.—and can be easily damaged. This is why you should never shake a baby.

Another difference is that a baby's nerves lack "squelching power". An adult's nerves have learned to deal with minor stimuli, to sort them out and to screen them. It's like a bouncer at a nightclub or a firewall on your computer—undesirables can be squelched before they ever get through the gate. In neurological terms, what keeps unimportant impulses out so the brain can concentrate on bigger issues is referred to as "threshold". When nerves get sufficient stimulation, the threshold is exceeded, allowing the nerve to transmit the stimulating impulse on up to the brain.

Newborn babies don't yet have their thresholds set. This is why subluxation can play such a huge role in the development of the harmful somatogastric reflex arcs and pathways detailed below. Some of these painful reflex arcs can wreak havoc.

THE BRAIN DELEGATES LEARNED PATTERNS TO THE SPINE

The spinal column is the largest proprioceptive structure in the body governing balance, spatial orientation, acceleration and movement. A baby's spine needs to learn how to balance and orient the body in a three dimensional world. This proprioceptive learning process begins near birth and it continues for years. Anything that interferes with it can cause problems. Some will be seen in the short term, others won't manifest until years later.

For a baby to learn good proprioceptive-, neuromuscular-, and cross-crawl patterning, several areas—primarily the eyes, ears, spine, skin, arms and legs—must all communicate well. The brain receives messages from all of these areas, then integrates this information and forms appropriate reflexes (for example, to contract certain muscles while relaxing others) in order to control and coordinating the whole process of "being in the world".

The brain does this constantly, with every movement and breath, every visual, aural and somatic stimulus. It takes a lot of time, trial and error and stored experiences before the new brain gets it right. When crawling is finally achieved without loss of balance or banging into things, the brain gets bored with running the whole proprioceptive show. Then it does what any good boss does; it delegates that whole complex set of learned reactions to the spinal cord. This frees up billions of neurons in the brain, so baby can use them for more important stuff, like learning to say, "Hi Mom, luv ya!"

After a pattern of behavior is delegated to the cord, it essentially becomes permanent behavior that is very difficult to change. So, if a baby remains subluxated long enough, aberrant neuropathic cycles may go from the brain to the cord, effectively locking those cycles into the child's behavior patterns. Like riding a bike, once the cord learns a pattern, it won't be forgotten. That's one reason why chiropractors recommend early correction of subluxations in children; they need to be adjusted before the aberrant neuropathies can centralize.

THE ROLE OF THE VAGUS NERVE (CN 10)

Chiropractors have long felt that subluxation at the atlas can have a dramatic affect on the tenth cranial (vagus) nerve and on the function of the organs it supplies. This is especially so with babies, presumably because their brain stem extends into the upper cervical spine. Adjusting that is specific to the upper cervical spine (Atlas/Axis) very often improves visceral function for the organs that are supplied by CN 10—from the head down to the liver. Thus, this nerve controls the swallowing reflex, peristalsis, respiration, heart rate, stomach acid, duodenal function, etc.

I think that upper cervical subluxation at birth is why we see so many babies under the bilirubin lights in hospitals for several days at a time—CN 10 is affected, and the liver grows sluggish and has trouble eliminating surplus red blood cells. These surplus cells turn the baby orangish-yellow, and the bili lights are the standard treatment. My personal observation of the babies I've adjusted shortly after birth is that they rarely show such yellowing, and if they do, it's slight and of short duration. This leads me to conclude that chiropractic care has a beneficial effect on visceral function in neonates.

A personal experience supports this conclusion. In January 1976, when I was a student at Palmer College of Chiropractic, a classmate's wife delivered their first baby in a local hospital. The infant immediately began having problems and kept getting worse. First diagnosed as liver damage, the situation developed into what is now called "Failure to Thrive". Despite IV feeding and the finest medical care in the Midwest, by the fourth week he had lost over 30% of his birth weight and was on life support. Mike, my classmate, asked permission to bring in a teaching chiropractor to check his son's spine. Predictably, the hospital denied his request. (In Davenport there was a great deal of conflict between chiropractors and medicine, as the famous Wilk et al. v. AMA et al. lawsuit was in progress at that time.) The hospital actually obtained a court injunction preventing Mike from seeing his dying son, on the grounds that the baby was under hospital care and since he was in critical condition, any chiropractic treatment might kill him!

Mike was a devoted father. He also played on the rugby team. Faced with the injunction, he took immediate action. He organized the whole Rugby team, some of the toughest and strongest men in the Midwest, to go to the hospital en masse, taking with them one of the finest chiropractors in Davenport. Easily pushing the doctors aside, they forced their way into the intensive care ward, where three Rugby players barred the door while the senior chiropractor examined Mike's baby. He found a raging spinal subluxation at Atlas and quickly adjusted it. Then the team left just as fast as they had arrived. Before the police could get to the hospital, the baby's vital signs had begun to improve, and within a week he returned to normal birth weight and was discharged ... as "healthy"!

I have no doubt if the Rugby team hadn't made possible that one precisely placed upper cervical specific adjustment (Gonstead listing ASR, by the way), Mike's baby would have died. I don't say this lightly, and I base my opinion upon two things and two things only. First, the baby began to die as soon as he was born, and he showed absolutely no improvement in spite of intensive, expert medical care. His vitals deteriorated steadily, his body continued to lose weight and his doctors grew increasingly worried. Second, the baby made a dramatic turnaround immediately after receiving his adjustment. There was no other viable explanation for the recovery; no new miracle drugs or treatments had been administered. The only new variable introduced into the equation was the chiropractic adjustment. The only logical conclusion is that the adjustment saved his life.

NERVE HARMONY

Your car has controls to give it gas, steer it, make it stop. In order to drive, you need each of these controls to work in perfect harmony or you wouldn't make it very far without causing a wreck. The human nerve system also has many interactive controls. The sympathetic and parasympathetic nerves tell the organs, respectively, to speed up or slow down. They act much like a car's gas and brake pedals and must work in perfect unimpinged harmony in order for optimal health to prevail.

As in a car, the "gas" and "brake" nerves work in synchronous opposition; when the brain wants an organ to speed up, it sends inhibitory impulses down the parasympathetic nerves and it sends stimulatory impulses down the sympathetic nerves. If either of these messages gets scrambled, it's rather like stomping on the gas and the brake at the same time—both start to wear out fast!

Lasting good health comes only from a well-harmonized interaction among these and other nerves. If disharmony exists, the target organ begins to malfunction. With continued malfunction, homeostatic parameters become breeched and illness appears. For example, if the pancreas is affected by a subluxation, its secretion rates can be artificially accelerated or retarded, leading to abnormally high or low blood sugar levels. A neuropathic event such as this and many others can occur more easily in the newborn, whose nerve system is particularly susceptible to badly scrambled inputs. By restoring proper neural flow, spinal adjusting restores a newborn's neural harmony … and when harmony is restored, optimal health soon returns.

TROPHIC SUPPLY / AXOPLASMIC FLOW

Chiropractors have been claiming since the latter days of the nineteenth century that in addition to the basic nerve impulse (which is electrical), there is also a vital impulse (which is intelligent) that is conveyed via our 32 pairs of spinal nerves. This vital impulse, chiropractors assert, is absolutely crucial to optimum health and homeostasis. These early chiropractors didn't know what to call it, but they suspected that it was there. A few decades later, technology caught up with their theories and supplied a name.

In the 1970s researchers tagged proteins with radioisotopes and injected them into rats in order to map the paths these proteins would travel. They expected the proteins to go to the brain and lodge there, which they did. Then the amazed researchers watched them travel down the spinal cord and easily cross the dural sleeve (the membrane where the spinal nerves leave the spine) then flow down the axons all the way to the organs. The dural sleeve was thought to be an "impenetrable" barrier (the so-called blood-brain barrier) and crossing it was considered the biological equivalent to walking though prison bars.

The scientists had discovered "trophic supply" or "axoplasmic flow", the "something more" those early twentieth century chiropractors had posited as flowing along spinal nerves.

As explanations were called for, the scientists concluded that this was some form of neurochemical communication wherein certain proteins, amino acids, etc., actually flow from the brain along the nerves to an organ, conveying some type of message. Since the organs tend to grow and function better when these nerves are intact, the term trophic (i.e. relating to nutrition) supply came into vogue. Since babies are rapidly growing, it stands to reason that proper trophic supply means even more to a baby's health than to an adult's.

To grasp trophic supply, think about the borderline digestive process in a quadriplegic whose spinal cord has been severed and compare it to the dynamic digestive process of a marathon runner. The former has only autonomic nerve supply to the gut; the latter has a fully interactive neural supply, including trophic supply, from intact spinal nerve root communication.

SOMATOVISCERAL AND VISCEROSOMATIC REFLEXES

There are numerous reflexes at work in a baby. A pediatrician examines a few of these when assessing newborns. One of these is the Babinski Reflex, which is elicited by firmly stroking the sole of the foot, if the reflex is present, it is predictive of certain nerve system diseases in adulthood. The Fencer Reflex is triggered by gently turning a sleeping baby's head to one side and holding it there. Soon, the baby's arms will go into the classic posture of a poised fencer. These commonly-tested-for reflexes are indicative only of rare neurological problems and are of little use to parents. One other reflex, however, holds more meaning, and if you understand a little bit about it, your job as a parent becomes easier.

A Somatovisceral Reflex (SVR) starts in the body (soma) and then involves an internal organ (viscera). It is hypothesized as a cause of colic (dubbed a "somatogastric reflex"). Most SVRs occur in response to sharp, unexpected pain somewhere on the body. For infants, this could be a sharp pain such as a needle prick in the foot to draw blood or circumcision. It could also be due to spinal subluxation. But wherever the pain occurs, the SVR provides bad input to a target organ. Simply put, an outer part of the body hurts, and an internal organ suffers for it. A baby's fairly blank (i.e. undeveloped) nerve system has little experience in processing pain. Some of the pain impulses go haywire, and instead of going up the spinal cord directly to the brain, they take a detour and arrive at an internal organ. Once there, the aberrant impulse creates disharmony. A reflex pathway is thus born. In the case of colic, the Somatovisceral Reflex affects the gastrointestinal tract causing gas, pain, reversed peristalsis, poor assimilation of foodstuffs, etc. Hospital births are loaded with painful events that can easily initiate a somatovisceral reflex.

The AMA has known about somatovisceral reflexes for decades. In November 1958, H. Kamieth, MD, published a study in the *Journal of the American Medical Association* detailing his findings after x-raying 100 ulcer patients. He found a very high correlation between thoracic spine misalignments and ulcers, noting that when the spine was misaligned to the left, the ulcer was in the stomach, when misaligned to the right, the ulcer was in the duodenum. These observations illustrate the chiropractic principle that soma and viscera are indeed related.

In 1979, at Anaheim, California, I attended an interdisciplinary conference on the spine. Among the many famous scientists who spoke was Akio Sato, MD, of Japan, who had studied the SVR for decades. In one experiment, Dr. Sato studied gastric acid motility in cats. He documented that by merely placing an ice cube on the cat's skin, its stomach acid level changed reflexively within seconds! Imagine that, a somatic stimulus affecting stomach acid. Are we talking "colic" yet?

(The flip side to the SVR is the Viscerosomatic Reflex, in which an internal organ malfunctions, thus sending aberrant neural input to the outside aspect of the body. This reflex is chronic and does not affect infants or children—they haven't lived long enough to manifest it. As examples of the VSR: ovarian cysts can refer pain to the spine, particularly the low back; angina refers to the left arm; temporomandibular joint (TMJ) troubles refer pain to the face, neck or scalp, and so on.)

So, there you have an introduction to infant neurology. We know that the nerves affect the organs. We know that spinal subluxation affects the nerves. And we know that all of the nerves must work in perfect harmony in order to have a healthy, happy baby. Lastly, we postulate that by adjusting subluxation, neural harmony is restored and then you get a happy baby.

CHIROPRACTIC'S ROLE FOR COLICKY BABIES

The very first colic study that I read was done about 1995 at Palmer College of Chiropractic-West, in Sunnyvale, California, I believe. The study split colicky babies into two groups; one group received chiropractic adjustments twice per week, the other received a sham manipulation but no specific vertebral adjustment. Chiropractic students performed these adjustments under the close supervision of senior instructing chiropractors. Initially, these babies cried on average five hours per day. The exit survey revealed that the sham group experienced no reduction in crying time. The group receiving chiropractic care cut crying time in half. I remember that those facts angered me because if a chiropractic adjustment was done properly, the crying should have been <u>gone</u> by the end of the survey period!

Reading the case histories in this book, you may notice that none of the babies is reported as having the same subluxation. For some, spinal subluxation in the middle back can trigger colic. For others, it might be the neck or even cranial faults. I'm convinced that this is one reason this study reduced only half the crying. All the treatment was aimed at the same exact spot on every baby. It's a common error when science tries to research chiropractic. Chiropractic is focused upon balancing the whole body—it is not a one size fits all assembly line but a calling that recognizes that people are individuals, with widely varying spinal and biomechanical needs.

Granted, students were doing the adjusting for this study, and that would not have been as effective as using doctors experienced the field. I should be glad that the babies at least got partial relief, but I wish they hadn't published that flawed result as if it were something to brag about, for students and practitioners both might interpret such a low bar as the standard for patient care. If graduating chiropractors think 50 percent improvement is a valid goal, my fear is that before long, the bar will be lowered again, and eventually failure to eliminate colic becomes the norm. Should that point arrive, new chiropractors may join the allopaths in singing "Colic's Incurable ... Colic is Normal!"

I repeat, most colic is totally "curable" with just a few specific chiropractic adjustments. The technique has been so successful for me that I cannot even imagine just a 50 percent improvement. My toughest case to date, in January 2006, required four visits over 17 days. On her first visit, the infant's arms and legs were drawn tightly up against her body and her reddened face was deeply wrinkled by pain as she cried non-stop. On her last visit, I adjusted her by gently coaxing the last cranial bone into place as she breast-fed. Her body was loose and relaxed as she slept, and her look was one of total bliss. That's how babies should be ... blissful, and it is chiropractic's role to return them to that natural, blissful state.

FROM MY FILES—JANUARY 2006:

Nathaniel had colic and a huge, deformed head. At eleven months old he looked like an alien from space. He had had a suction cup delivery. Doctors had diagnosed too much cerebrospinal fluid inside the skull and had scheduled Nathaniel for surgery to put shunts in his brain to balance the CSF pressure.

This intrigued me, because one of the theories we had learned in Sacro Occipital Technique involved unbalanced CSF pressures and here was a child with just such a problem!

I asked Julie to bring him in for evaluation, figuring, "What do we have to lose? He's already scheduled for surgery." I discovered a subluxation at C1 and adjusted him. He cried so loudly that it scared me. Julie tried to reassure me by saying, "Oh, he can cry even louder than that!"

Two weeks later, all signs of Nathaniel's formerly huge misshapen head were gone. His doctors cancelled the surgery and called it a miracle. I call it an adjustment. Julie reported that he began crawling with his head held up. Before his adjustment, he crawled with his head hanging down, never looking where he was going. It had probably hurt too much to look up! (Atlas subluxation. Two adjustments, one week apart. Colic gone after first week. Head regained normal shape in ten days.)

CHAPTER 4

FINDING A BABY-FRIENDLY CHIROPRACTOR

CHIROPRACTIC USES NO DRUGS

I need to emphasize that chiropractors are drugless practitioners. We don't think in terms of drugs, we don't talk drugs and we don't prescribe drugs. If you happen upon a chiropractor who is eager to discuss drugs, my advice is to run away—you're talking to a "wannabe MD" not a dedicated chiropractor.

CHIROPRACTIC IS "OPERATOR DEPENDENT"

I also need to reiterate something that we chiropractors don't really like to mention—not all chiropractors are equally skilled. Our technical skills vary from one practitioner to the next, and in this respect chiropractic is unlike medicine. You might switch from one medical doctor to another, and you'll probably find the same basic set of medical skills (barring specialties) in all of them. This doesn't necessarily hold true with chiropractic care, in spite of what you might hear to the contrary, and this disparity can affect the level of care your baby will receive.

I find it odd that most patients won't hesitate to get a second medical opinion, especially if the problem is grave or the first MD's treatment isn't effective. But when it comes to chiropractors, the public tends to lump us all together. When one DC fails to get results, the patient tends to gives up on chiropractic altogether. It always makes me sad to hear that, because I know that a second chiropractor could make all the difference in the outcome. I love chiropractic; I'm proud of what it can do when used properly. Unfortunately, it is not always used specifically or properly.

THE BEST WAY TO LOCATE A GOOD DC

At this point, I want to walk you through the process of locating and interviewing a chiropractor for your baby. This overview should be particularly helpful for anyone who has had no prior experience with chiropractic. But I want to say first that there's a much faster way to find a "good one" than following the steps I will outline. Ask people who've taken their own babies to a chiropractor for a recommendation. If they had a good experience, they will probably be eager to talk about it.

Most young parents are less nervous if they already know that I helped their friends' babies. Once you've seen someone else's baby get well, you naturally are more inclined to have your baby adjusted. It becomes easier to think of a chiropractic solution once you talk to others who have already achieved that.

TIPS FOR SURFING THE YELLOW PAGES

If you cannot get a word-of-mouth recommendation, I suggest that you get a pen and open the yellow pages to chiropractors. Please draw a big X through the largest ads. The biggest ads sometimes promote the worst adjusters, who must attract a high volume of new patients just to pay for this very expensive advertising. It is likely that these DCs have hired high-priced professional practice consultants, whose focus is entirely upon helping the doctor increase his or her profit. There's nothing wrong with profit, but when it becomes the doctor's driving force, patient care goes out the window. In a nutshell, when you see a big ad, it's a great reason to look further.

DCs whose ads feature "The Eight (or Ten) Danger Signals" should also be avoided. Using fear to attract clients should have no place in chiropractic. I would also recommend that you X-out the ads promoting workers' compensation and personal injury cases. These doctors are unlikely to be interested in treating babies, though they may not say that to you at first.

The next candidates for deletion are the ads in which chiropractors try to mimic physicians. Experience has taught me that these emulators cannot perform adjustments well. You'll save yourself time, money and frustration by avoiding practitioners who advertise themselves as a "Chiropractic Physician". Under some state laws, a DC might be called "Chiropractic Physician", but I personally would be leery of a yellow page ad that said more than simply "Chiropractor" or "Doctor of Chiropractic".

In a large city, you'll still have dozens of ads to sort through after these initial deletions. You might want to cross out those that promote the doctor's specialty adjusting instruments, lasers, weight loss or other such issues. Such promotional fluff is designed to get more paying customers through the door, and none of this is needed or desired for adjusting babies.

SOME QUESTIONS TO ASK YOUR POTENTIAL NEW CHIROPRACTOR

When you've isolated a few likely candidates, I recommend calling each office. See how they answer the phone. Ask a few questions, and pay more attention to how your questions are answered than to the answers themselves. Listen carefully for rudeness or a defensive tone in the DC's voice, if you hear it, that person is probably to be avoided.

"Do you adjust infants?" You should hear a resounding "Yes!" from whomever you talk to, be it the DC or receptionist. (You may happen to get a receptionist who is new on the job and might be unused to this uncommon question. So don't judge too quickly if s/he just doesn't know.)

"Where did you go to chiropractic college?" The doctor should be eager to answer this one, and so should his or her staff. The answer is important. You may find this hard to believe, but some chiropractic colleges don't even teach adjusting technique! When I sat before the chiropractic licensing board in order to practice in Iowa in 1987, there was a young chiropractor sitting next to me who had graduated from a chiropractic college in Illinois, where he had been practicing for three years. He hit only one minor snag when seeking a license in Iowa; he hadn't taken a single class in adjusting technique! Imagine how foolish it would be if a dentist never had a classroom hour in drilling teeth or a surgeon had never seen a scalpel. (Amazingly, the young man was issued a temporary license, provided that within six months he take and pass just *one* course in Palmer technique, i.e how to detect and correct subluxations.)

Top U.S. schools that emphasize adjusting skills are Palmer (one each in Iowa, Florida and California), Logan (Missouri), and Life (Georgia and California). Doctors who graduated from other schools might well be effective, but those schools are not known for their emphasis on chiropractic adjusting technique. I'm perhaps the first DC to state this opinion in print, so don't expect others to agree with me. This is something no one in my profession likes to discuss openly.

Just because a doctor graduated at one of these other colleges doesn't necessarily make him or her a poor adjuster. Some doctors learn their adjusting skills after they begin practice and find that they are dissatisfied with their clinical results. Conversely, you might encounter a real loser who graduated from one the best schools. There are always exceptions.

There are a few chiropractic colleges that try to mimic medical schools in training and terminology. These colleges place zero to low priority on the technical aspects of specifically correcting subluxations. I have never figured out why they settle for training "wannabe" doctors of medicine. I have met three chiropractors that mimicked allopaths. None of them was a skilled adjuster. If you call such a person, you can probably pick up clues on the phone—they'll either deflect your questions away from specifics about adjustment technique or try to snow you with four-syllable words in medi-babble.

"When did you graduate?" Whenever I treat a patient who is visiting from out of town, I ask if they know when their hometown chiropractor graduated. The answer tells me which of my techniques to use. Because teaching chiropractic adjusting has lately become less important at chiropractic colleges (even in the top tier schools), the younger the chiropractor, the more limited will have been his or her instruction in effective, specific spinal adjusting technique. (Like me, you may find this state of affairs hard to imagine. In the late 1990s, several chiropractic colleges were sued. They reacted by increasing "risk management", i.e. it's better to teach less technique than to teach plenty and get sued for it. Now, young chiropractors are at an awesome disadvantage, when it comes to obtaining technical expertise—they must learn it after graduating!) As with the previous question, this one has qualifiers. An older field doctor may have sponsored a younger colleague and personally taught him or her the "good stuff". Likewise, there are some old coots who simply cannot adjust very well.

"Do you have children?" If the doctor has kids, that could be a major plus. In a word: they can feel your pain. When it comes to treating babies, I don't think book learning can substitute for direct, personal experience. Which is not to say that you should turn your back on a childless chiropractor who has treated babies successfully.

"Can I get a free consultation?" The answer should be yes. A free consult allows the doctor and the patient a little truce time, where each can get to know the other without too much commitment. I like doing free consults. They help me decide if I want to take a case or not because I don't like treating people I'm uncomfortable with or who are uncomfortable with me. If your request for a free consult is granted, you're looking at someone of like mind. Bear in mind, however, that free consultations are not for hours-long chatter. Chiropractors are busy. Ten minutes should be plenty.

"Can you provide references?" When entrusting your baby to a new type of doctor who uses new methods, you're entitled to ask for references. I have a list of patients who have given me permission to use them as references, and I generally provide the newcomer with two or three phone numbers. My patients do a better job of advertising than I could ever do.

"How long will it take?" If your baby's case is indeed a candidate for chiropractic care, it should take fewer than three weeks to address the colic. If you are given a very different answer, and especially if you are asked to sign a contract for a set number of treatments over a set period of time, I recommend that you find a different DC.

QUESTIONS THAT MAY SEEM IMPORTANT BUT ARE REALLY POINTLESS

Given how little time you will have to ask the important questions, I'd like to point out some that simply aren't worth asking of a chiropractor—although they may be pertinent for other professions.

"Are you a member of any professional organizations?" This may be an informative question if directed at an MD, but all a chiropractor has to do is send an organization a few hundred bucks and presto, s/he's a member in good standing. The organization may provide the DC with less expensive malpractice insurance, discounts on seminars and maybe a plaque for the wall, but it doesn't mean a thing for patient care and won't help your crying baby.

"Do you use 'light force'?" Some people have heard the term "light force" applied to chiropractic and may think it's important to use it when treating an infant. There are certain techniques associated with this term (also known as low force or non-force or instrument adjusting), most of which use a percussion-producing instrument to provide the thrust instead of using the hands. The problem with using such instruments is that it is easy to over adjust when using them—especially on an infant. Learning osseous force technique (i.e. manual adjusting) is difficult, but it is paramount that this be mastered in order to provide good chiropractic care—whether manually or with an instrument. Good technique is the issue here, not the amount of force applied. Besides, we are all gentle with an infant.

"Do you take x-rays?" Asking this of a DC is irrelevant to your immediate needs. Babies don't have much actual bone in their spines and what they do have shows up on x-ray only as tiny white spots. It takes many years of degeneration before a DC might see radiological evidence of a subluxation. If a DC tells you that X-rays are necessary before s/he will agree to treat your baby, keep searching!

THE MONEY QUESTION

Whether or not chiropractic care will be covered by your insurance shouldn't be a dominating factor in choosing a chiropractor for your baby. If you find someone you think will be a good match, go with that choice. Your baby will only need a few visits— most infants need only two or three to lose the colic. If the problem persists, there is something else going on. In mid 2009 I charge $60 per visit, most other DCs in this area charge comparable fees. Fees in major cities will be higher. Rather than ask about insurance, you might ask if a cash discount is available. It's common to see discounts of up to 20 percent offered if fees are paid in cash at the time of service. (Though it's beyond the scope of this book to discuss it in any detail, I feel compelled to mention that in insurance-driven practices, the practitioner has to dance to the tune that the insurance company plays, and this can have a drastic, negative impact on patient care. It's happening throughout the health care industry, and chiropractic is not exempt.)

THE CONSULTATION

As you first step into the office of the chiropractors you've pre-screened, use your senses and trust your feelings, beginning as soon as you twist the doorknob. Here are a few clues to note:

Office Smell. If it smells like wintergreen, incense or athletic balm, be suspicious! In my experience, offices that smell like balms almost always signal crude adjustors whose routine patients are so sore that they need analgesics! (Proficient, specific adjustors have little use for balms.)

Busy or Quiet? Don't be misled by either situation. The nature of chiropractic offices is such that "crowd density" varies by the hour. In addition, most doctors schedule free consults for times that aren't going to be too busy. That leaves us free to actually listen to you. An empty office may signal anything from good scheduling to a bad chiropractor with no patients. A crowded office may signal anything from bad scheduling to effective advertising to a really good chiropractor. It's hard to tell on an initial visit. Staff. Most DCs have a small staff. Quite a few actually have no staff at all. That's unlike medical offices, which need lots of personnel to handle the procedures, drugs, surgical instruments, records, lab tests, etc. So concentrate on assessing the degree of compassion and warmth you feel from the staff. If you feel at ease, you're probably in a good place.

The DC. Most good chiropractors are user-friendly and should be able to put you at ease. A good DC would rather listen than talk. The consult should be centered on you and your baby, not on the doctor touting his or her expertise, credentials or other superfluous issues. You should be getting good eye contact and careful attention during your interview.

The Fee Discussion. This should be clear and frank. I usually try to put the young parents at ease by saying right up front, "This consult is free. If you decide that you want me to treat your baby, I charge $60 for each visit, but there's no charge for this consult and there's no obligation." Then we get down to the actual consultation.

Contracts. I don't recommend signing any agreement for contract care, which is a rip-off, pure and simple. To my mind, contracts are a chiropractor's way of saying, "I am no good at what I do, so I need to lock you into a treatment plan." I like to think of chiropractic offices as restaurants—you try the food, and if you like it, you'll come back when you want more.

We are Drugless Practitioners. Unlike medical offices, where staff and doctor speak openly and freely about drugs, the chiropractic office will not do this. Don't be alarmed or turned off if your prospective DC. avoids discussing drugs. Knowledge of drugs is not a prerequisite for chiropractors; in fact, we are restricted by law from discussing drugs with patients. I have had a few new patients judge me harshly because I refused to discuss drugs with them. It would be a mistake to pass judgment on a drugless practitioner merely because he or she won't talk about drugs.

Your Assessment. By the end of the consultation, you should have some feel for the doctor—either you'll feel good or you'll keep looking. When you find the right DC, you'll be glad you took the time to shop around.

CHAPTER 5

YOUR BABY'S FIRST VISIT
TO THE CHIROPRACTOR

ENCOUNTERING PRE-VISIT RESISTANCE

Some women are surprised to encounter resistance when they say they're going to take the baby (or child) to a chiropractor. Sometimes, the arguments can get ugly. People who have negative opinions about chiropractic care for babies, might react more favorably if you said you were taking the baby to a witch doctor.

Resistance at Home.   Strong resistance rarely comes from the baby's father, who is usually so tired of the constant crying that he's likely to say, "Go for it ... whatever it takes!" They are ready to try anything that promises peace and quiet. The in-laws, however, are a likely source of opposition in my experience. If their stereotypical thinking limits the sphere of chiropractic to old people with old backs, it can be helpful to point out to them that a lot of those bad backs first developed in youth.

Resistance from the Medical Establishment. Your pediatrician may also rebel, perhaps strongly, against the idea of taking the baby to a chiropractor. Although some of the medical prejudice against chiropractic is slowly fading, it is still fairly common to find doctors who are against it. Remember Angie's story from the Preface to this book? Her pediatrician said he would no longer treat her baby if Angie took the child to a chiropractor. (For an in-depth look at the MDs' war against chiropractic, see the Chapter 9.) In spite of chiropractic's wonderful results with colic, I have yet to have a single case referred to me by a pediatrician.

The "chiropractic isn't for kids" mindset is deeply entrenched. In the early 1990s, chiropractic was finally approved for limited inclusion into certain military health insurance programs. However, in response to lobbying by the AMA power structure, U.S. government regulations make it a point to restrict military plans for chiropractic only to those over 18 years of age!

Psychological Resistance. Some women feel, or are made to feel, that they're doing a bad job as a mom if the baby has colic. They internalize the idea that if the baby doesn't get better in the predicted span of time, doesn't "grow out of it", it must be their fault; they must be doing something wrong. I can appreciate how painful it must be when someone insinuates that a young mother isn't doing it right. When the doctor says, "It's normal … relax! Your baby will grow out of it," the implication is that she can't even handle a "normal" problem. This can wreak emotional havoc on her, bringing up emotions of guilt and shame—even though the colic is not her fault.

The new mother's own mom or friends can also do more harm than good. A patient once told me, "My best friend came over, and after ten minutes of listening to my baby crying, she got up and left. I followed her outside and she said, 'Oh, that crying's not so bad.' It's easy to say that when it's not your baby!"

Feelings of self blame are likely to make the mother even more harried and depressed, which can lead to a feeling of fatalism, a conviction that nothing can be done about colic that hasn't been done. And since what has been done hasn't worked, it's all her fault and no other external efforts (and she's tried them all) will work.

RESPONDING TO THE RESISTANCE

The most important element in mustering your forces to respond to the resistance is to remember and believe that the mother is not at fault and is not to blame. Self confidence makes it easier to weather a storm of resistance. In many cases, calm and reasoned arguments will turn the tide. Show the person in question this book, enlist the cooperation of a friend whose child has been treated successfully, take the high road. However, there may be times when it feels as if you're talking to a brick wall. Here are some alternatives:

Opt not to use Chiropractic. If the pressure against seeing a DC is too great, it might save your marriage to let your baby cry until the colic goes away by itself. Remember that the medical websites agree that the common treatment option is no treatment.

Make the "Put Up Or Shut Up" Challenge. The loudest boos always come from the free seats. You might suggest that the critics agree to take care of your baby until the colic goes away.

Understand That Silence Is Golden. Some mothers choose to see a DC on the sly, without telling anyone. By the time others find out, the baby's completely better. You have the right to do whatever it takes to help your baby, and that includes keeping silent.

WHAT TO EXPECT AT THE OFFICE

Unlike an adult patient, a baby can't tell me where it hurts. I can and do get information from the mother, but for the most part, I rely on my fingertips and years of training and experience. The initial exam includes quite a bit of gentle palpating to look for signs of subluxation. Palpation is a series of light touches, sometimes with a slight amount of pressure, over and around key points on the baby's body. It's a diagnostic tool that can reveal taut and tender muscle fibers, altered sweat gland activity, porous or closed skin cells, tender points, muscle tone and temperature differences between the left and right sides of the body. We also look for small areas of the skin that feel different from adjacent areas. It's hard to describe this sensation or to demonstrate it to someone who hasn't yet developed sufficient tactile sensitivity. This is not magic or voodoo; it's more like reading Braille, an ability that develops only with proper training and diligent, motivated practice. With palpation, chiropractors have been reading the "Braille" on bodies for a long time.

Occasionally, a patient will remark that a doctor, physical therapist, etc. had done what seemed like palpation and "couldn't feel anything". Please take it to heart when I emphasize that only chiropractors have the proper training to find subluxations, and it takes years to learn to detect them. It is not a skill other practitioners are trained in, and without the training, it can't be done ... just like reading Braille.

At chiropractic college and in the many years since, I've taken several courses and seminars that included specific techniques for use with infants and children ... commonly referred to as "baby technique". (These are listed in detail in "About the Author" at the end of this book.) Baby technique means how to tailor the analysis, adjustment and force used to "fit" the size of the patient, as well as how to integrate normal pediatric concerns into the analysis. Every patient is different, and how I would adjust your baby will probably be different from how I would adjust your sister's baby.

So you can get a feel for what it might be like when your baby is in the office, let me give you an example. Assume that after palpation, I've discovered that the baby's atlas is subluxated. If it were the mother's atlas, I would place her face down on the adjusting table, adjust the tension and position of the table and headrest to reflect her height, weight and the three dimensional nature of the subluxation, and then I would perform the adjustment. I don't do any of that with a baby whose atlas is subluxated.

To adjust a baby's atlas, I have the mother hold the baby in her arms so they're face to face, and I ask her to lie on her back on the adjusting table with the baby resting on her chest. This has several advantages for all concerned—both of my hands are free to examine and treat the baby, the baby is secure in the mother's arms (a soothing position), and the mother can feel exactly how light the pressure is that I apply when making the adjustment.

Other adjustments, such as thoracic, lumbar or cranial, for example, can be done while the mother sits in a chair holding the baby.

WILL THE ADJUSTMENT CAUSE YOUR BABY PAIN?

In a single word: No. The adjustment won't cause pain, but your baby might cry anyway. Some babies have already experienced scary and painful medical procedures, and so when the chiropractor starts gently probing, some babies are primed to start screaming. This is a defense mechanism; the only one a baby has!

In general, when treating babies I hope there's an alternative to treating them when they're crying. Sometimes that's not possible in the case of colic, but whenever possible, I want to examine and adjust babies while they are sleeping or breast-feeding. The fact that they rarely wake up or stop nursing when I make the adjustment tells me that the specific vertebral adjustment is not painful. In fact, it's quite common to see a look of calm or a smile sweep across the baby's face at the moment of adjustment.

CHAPTER 6

AFTER THE ADJUSTMENT: FOLLOW UP VISITS AND AVOIDING "RELAPSE"

Most of the time, a baby stops crying between one and ten minutes after the adjustment. Some babies initially cry a bit more after their adjustment, although parents tell me that the tone of the crying is much less desperate or agonized. Most commonly the baby starts to relax and stretch out, maybe even coos. It always makes me feel good to see such a wonderful transformation and to know that I played a part in it.

ARE FOLLOW UP VISITS NEEDED?

I really want to see a baby for a follow-up visit, and your chiropractor probably will too. I can't wait to see that smile again, but there's also another reason to reschedule. Adjusting is an art. We're trying to move vertebrae back into precise alignment and optimal function, and we're doing it through several layers of tissue. It might take a few days to determine whether we merely reduced the subluxation or if we corrected it completely.

In my practice, I stop treating as soon as the subluxation is corrected and the baby gets blissful. I believe that babies have better things to do than keep seeing me. So, when the crying's all gone, the baby stays home. Other chiropractors have different opinions on follow-up strategies.

PRESERVING THE ADJUSTMENT: PROPER BABY-HANDLING TECHNIQUE

Once your baby's spine is aligned correctly, you'll want to preserve the adjustment with good baby handling technique because a baby can be re-subluxated, and the initial symptoms or different symptoms may appear as a consequence. So, the first order of business is to make sure that a subluxation doesn't recur. Proper handling isn't particularly difficult and it will provide a lifetime of positive feedback for your child.

<u>Support the Head</u>. Some babies become subluxated due to improper handling during their first few weeks. Until an infant has the muscular development to support his or her

head unaided, anyone who picks up your baby should put one hand under the butt and the other hand should cradle the head to support the baby when lifting. This technique protects the baby against subluxation.

Avoid Sustained Upright Positions. The sling/wedge, "Johnny Jump-ups" and other devices that prematurely force young spines into partially upright positions will put a baby at risk for spinal damage. The damage from these devices may not show up until years later, when spinal scoliosis, bowed legs and hip problems begin to surface. It's wise to keep your infant horizontal as much as possible. When a baby lies on its tummy, it encourages development of the all-important neck muscles, and it promotes the formation of the normal, healthy cervical curve. This position also prompts babies to begin crawling, which is a crucial developmental stage. When your baby can sit up naturally, s/he is finally ready for short sessions in those upright devices. Until then, there is nothing to be gained by placing your baby in them; I recommend against it.

Schedule Lots of "Crawl Time". Today's babies are more often confined to car seats, strollers, cribs and other instruments of restraint than in previous generations. While some confinement is necessary, too much retards development, and I think most babies experience too much confinement. Babies who are allowed to crawl, roam, explore and take risks have been proven to show developmental advantages—they are more outgoing, courageous, and intelligent than their more confined counterparts. Kids that bypass the critical crawling phase end up at a mental and physical disadvantage. We know that crawling and other physical activity is vital to social, physical and mental well being.

<u>Note the Signals that Baby Needs "Maintenance Care"</u>. There are several clues that can alert parents that their baby may need an adjustment. The most common signs are changes in behavior, eating habits or sleep habits or when a normally active baby suddenly becomes much less active. A lack of symmetry in the face or torso can also be a clue, as can crying when you touch a specific body part. I usually sum up my advice on this by saying, "If your baby becomes unhappy, see me." I'm referring here to basic behavior change, however, not the routine squawks and fuss about diaper changes, etcetera. After

you see the "before and after" once or twice, you'll know what to look for.

Chiropractic care is great for babies and kids. I advise regular checkups to ensure that they remain free of subluxation. For people who wonder why kids need chiropractic checkups, I recommend observing children when they're hard at play. It won't take long to see that spinal care is a good idea!

It's better to stay well than to have to get well.

CHAPTER 7

WHAT IF CHIROPRACTIC DOESN'T HELP?

The curves Mother Nature throws us keep life interesting, but they definitely make the chiropractor's job harder! Although statistics show that chiropractic is effective in nine out of ten cases, some babies are still left crying. Let's hypothetically assume the worst, that your baby is among the still-miserable group and ask, "What are the next steps?"

1. <u>Make sure it's colic</u>! Pediatricians rarely make mistakes with this diagnosis, but it happens. Consider getting a second pediatrician's opinion to rule out causes other than colic. Since chiropractic works so well for colic, and since it didn't work in your case, please be alert to other medical issues.

2. <u>It may be time to change chiropractors</u> if the second pediatric opinion confirms colic. You might have picked someone who just wasn't up to the task. As mentioned earlier, Chiropractic is a science, a philosophy, and an art.

Just as no two artists will create exactly the same painting or sculpture, no two chiropractors will bring precisely the same artistic talents to a case. I have been amazed at seminars to see how wide a range of skills was on display, ranging from the brilliant to the pathetic. Indeed, the most inept practitioners might be popular and highly successful in business despite their level of technical skill. So I would always recommend finding another DC; although asking the first chiropractor for a referral might be ill advised, as s/he might well respond by trying to convince you that all your baby needs is additional treatment from the original source. If your baby hasn't improved in the first few sessions, there's no chance that more treatment from the same person will help. If the second DC brings no relief, go to step #3.

3. <u>Switch brands if you are feeding formula.</u> Formula is commonly mentioned as a possible cause of colic, so the observation must have some merit. One Finnish study surveyed kids with food allergies at age seven to nine; most had been colicky babies. Working backward from this finding, perhaps colic in that one out of ten babies who don't respond to chiropractic suggests an incompatibility with certain food elements or ingredients. A

masseuse once told me that she had been a colicky, bottle-fed baby whose colic disappeared when she was switched from formula to goat's milk.

4. <u>Switch to a low-flow nipple if you are feeding formula</u>. So-called "easy flow" nipples can worsen colic because too much formula floods the stomach all at once and dilutes the gastric acid. This surplus formula then sits and ferments, creating excess gas, noxious metabolic byproducts and pain. Babies' stomachs are designed for breast milk. In order to obtain breast milk, a baby has to suck fairly hard, and even with hard sucking, breast milk is released in a trickle, in perfect synchrony with the capacity of a tiny gut. Baby's fairly hard and regular sucking action is vital to healthy development of the swallow reflex. It also corrects cranial faults and stimulates the pineal gland, releasing growth hormones and endorphins. Suckling tonifies the throat and the Eustachian tubes in the ears and creates good dental arches. These are just some of the benefits of breast-feeding. Mothers who use formula can supply <u>some</u> of the benefits of breast-feeding simply by switching to a restricted nipple. Your baby will have to suck harder and longer to get a full belly. That alone might reduce colic.

5. <u>Change *your* diet if you're breast-feeding</u>. Certain foods make mother's milk taste bad. (The La Leche League nearest you will have full details.) You would be amazed at how quickly a "trigger" food can affect the flavor of your milk. My dad once kept dairy goats and produced the best goats' milk I've ever tasted. It sold out every day and people clamored for more. One day, people stopped buying it. He made me taste it and it was so undrinkable that even his dogs spurned it! Pop called the University of California at Davis, which mailed him the results of a study that tested the effect of various odors on cows' and goats' milk. The odors were passed before the animals' noses as they were being milked and each squirt of milk went into a labeled test tube. The results of subsequent double blind taste results showed that certain foods dramatically affected the milk's taste within seconds! My dad saw "wet straw" on the list of suspects, checked his barn and found that leaking rainwater had soured the bedding straw. He fixed the leak, changed the straw, and soon the milk was as sweet as ever, though he never did get back all of his customers. One glass of bad goats' milk will have that effect!

My point is that you could be eating (or inhaling) something that affects breast milk. That study was on goats and cows, but it certainly applies to all mammals. A case in point: a baby cried violently when nursing at home but nursed happily when the family went on vacation. Returning home, they discovered black mold around the windowsills, which apparently had a bad affect on the mother's milk. It might be wise to give some thought to the odors around you and your baby—deodorants, hair sprays, colognes, body washes, household chemicals and cleaning supplies, etc. Who can say which of these might be the culprit?

6. If you are breast-feeding, get an adjustment for yourself. Apparently, subluxations in the mother can affect breast milk in ways some babies can detect, be it quality or taste or something else. I've seen three cases in which the baby's colic remained until the mother got adjusted. While so few cases hardly qualify as a study, I've noticed that a few other DCs, reporting on chiropractic websites, have observed the same dramatic results.

7. Check out the home environment. Babies pick up on stress at home much more than you might imagine. If

there is marital stress or discord, your baby feels it. It could be why your baby has colic. Fumes, toxins, house mold and some pets may also be stressors for the baby. If you can't spot a culprit, consider asking your chiropractor or doctor to visit your house for a spot check by a fresh set of eyes.

8. <u>Do nothing.</u> If you've tried everything I just listed and still have a crying baby, consider waiting it out rather than try the risky approaches I list next. Doing nothing may sound contrary to what I've proposed thus far, but remember the first rule of medicine: "First, do no harm."

RISKY BUSINESS:
APPROACHES I WOULD NOT RECOMMEND

<u>Keeping the Baby Upright</u>. Some remedies are so new, so bizarre or so in conflict with science as to be considered risky. I put into this category the bands, the slings and the wedges often recommended for calming a crying baby. All of these put unnatural loads and premature strains on your baby's delicate spinal tissues, and, while they may seem like they're helping in the short term—the crying

slows down or stops— they can cause harm in the long term.

I'm convinced that putting your infant on a foam wedge, in a sling or doorway bouncer is tantamount to putting your baby on the rack. Especially during the first three months of life, babies have no business being seated in a partially upright position for extended periods of time—especially without full-body support.

The problem these devices cause has to do with the "Heuter-Volkman Phenomenon". When growing bone is subjected to mechanical stress, tiny electrical currents are generated that alter bone growth patterns. It takes just four or five minutes for the signals to trigger bone growth and the effect lasts for several hours. Placing an infant in an upright or partially upright position causes strains and generates electrical currents in the spine that send inappropriate growth messages to the eager young bones long after the baby has been relieved of the strain.

Given enough time and repetition, the upright position may initiate the abnormal spinal curvature called scoliosis. In chiropractic circles, such devices are thought to be a causative factor in the rising incidence of scoliosis, which was fairly rare in generations past. The surge in scoliosis seems to dovetail with the increased use of upright devices (and increased confinement). Rather than use these devices, keep your baby horizontal as much as possible and try to endure the crying—its adverse effects are not as long-term or as harmful as the damage an upright posture and the devices can inflict.

Administering Drugs or Antacids. It is beyond the scope of chiropractors to give advice about drugs. In fact, the average person on the street can tell you more about drugs than we legally can. But it doesn't take a genius to conclude that five-week-old babies shouldn't be drugged for a self-limiting problem like colic. Given that the medical experts agree that colic will go away by itself, why disturb your baby's delicate homeostatic balance?

The use of antacids to calm colic is contrary to the laws of biology. Like adults, babies are supposed to have acid in their stomachs. Acid helps break down food so that it can be assimilated. When stomach acid is inadequate, some proteins don't get broken down sufficiently, which causes the baby's immune system to treat them as antigens and attack them. Presto—your baby has developed the beginnings of a lifelong food allergy. Another function of stomach acid is to disable germs. If the acid isn't strong enough to do this, infection and/or disease may follow. Antacids rob your baby of the normal, natural, desirable level of gastric acid.

Diluting baby's stomach acid, thus lowering gastric pH, by administering excessive liquids is almost as harmful as neutralizing them with antacids. The easy-flow nipples are a common source of excessive liquid intake and should be avoided.

Before giving drugs to your infant, I invite you to look up the drug in the Physician's Desk Reference (PDR, available in libraries, clinics and, for a fee, online). It contains most of the current knowledge regarding drugs available to Western medicine and lists each drug's indications, contraindications and reported side effects. It is fairly common to look up a drug your child is taking and discover that it has side effects that exactly define his/her main health problem. It is also not uncommon to discover that the drug you've looked up is contraindicated for a given age group or condition. Watching a discussion of

Ritalin on Montel Williams' TV talk show, I heard one of the guests, a leading pediatrician, say that it's common practice for doctors to ignore the PDR age and dosage recommendations for Ritalin and other drugs. According to the PDR, Ritalin is only for children over six years of age; yet these physicians admitted on the air to routinely giving it to three-year-olds. Some doctors do this so routinely that they have a name for it —"Off-label" prescribing. Perhaps such information should make you as uneasy as it makes me. It never hurts to have information, and the PDR is a valuable source.

CHAPTER 8

BREAST-FEEDING:
A GREAT PREVENTATIVE

I have always maintained that the obvious mental and physical advantages breast-fed children enjoy are unmistakable. I can unequivocally assert that breast-fed babies suffer from colic much less often than formula fed babies. For decades pediatricians asserted that formula was "almost the equivalent" of breast milk, but in June 2007 the American Academy of Pediatricians (AAP) officially changed its tune and published its position paper on "Breast-feeding and the Use of Human Milk", which can be viewed at http://www.aap.org/policy/re9729.html.

The AAP policy states categorically that "Human milk is uniquely superior for infant feeding and is species-specific; all substitute feeding options differ markedly from it." It goes on to list the "compelling advantages to infants, mothers, families, and society from breast-feeding," including "health, nutritional, immunologic, developmental, psychological, social, economic and environmental benefits." These advantages include decrease in the incidence and/or severity of acute and chronic diseases, including diarrhea; a "possible protective effect" against additional diseases, many of them related to the digestive tract; and "possible enhancement of cognitive development". There appear to be almost as many benefits to the mother who breast-feeds, including easier and quicker recovery and improved bone remineralization postpartum as well as reduced risk of ovarian cancer and premenopausal breast cancer.

The AAP recommends that breast-feeding begin as soon as possible, usually within an hour after birth, and that exclusive breast-feeding will support optimal growth and development for approximately the child's first six months, during which time "other foods are generally unnecessary". So there you have the AAP official position. I would characterize it as an incentive to breast-feed!

I've noted a further health advantage for infants who breast-feed. A growing numbers of babies are having Eustachian tube surgery for recurring ear infections, and I'll bet that the vast majority of them are bottle-fed. Bottle-feeding does not require muscular effort on the baby's part, so the ear and throat complex don't get exercised, setting the stage for middle ear problems. Breast-feeding help to develop and tone the posterior oropharynx, the Eustachian structures and the other tissues that make for a healthy eye, ear, nose and throat. Babies I've observed being bottle-fed on plane flights frequently cry (or scream) on descent, while babies I've seen being breast-fed (including my own children) usually sleep peacefully or nurse during descent.

CHIROPRACTIC MAY HELP BABIES WHO HAVE TROUBLE NURSING

Babies with "dysfunctional nursing" have been shown to respond to chiropractic care. The *Journal of Clinical Chiropractic Pediatrics* (Vol. 4, No. 1, 1999) reports on two case studies where two infants were able to breast-feed normally after chiropractic care. An eight-week-old girl and four-week-old boy, both of whom had been unable to suckle properly since birth, were able to breast-feed normally after receiving chiropractic adjustments. Follow up showed that both continued to feed well.

FROM MY FILES—APRIL 2004:

Tiffany cried, on average, four hours a day, seven days a week. She was six months old and had been delivered in breech presentation. I found three subluxations. Two were between the shoulders; the other was in the extreme low back; a rare combination. I adjusted Tiffany, and she started cooing.

The next day she was still crying like crazy, but it sounded as though she were hungry. I checked Tiffany and no further adjustments were indicated. On a hunch, I asked Terri, "How's your milk?" She shrugged and said, "Oh, she doesn't seem to want my milk."

I asked Terri to get on the table, because in some cases, maternal subluxation affects milk. I found two that Terri's sacrum and second thoracic vertebra were subluxated. I adjusted Terri and said, "Go home and nurse your baby in an hour." It takes about an hour for the milk to change back.

Terri called me three hours later to say, "She's eating like a pig!" No wonder; her milk finally tasted good! (Tiffany: T3, T6, sacrum. One treatment. Zero colic after her first adjustment. Terri: T2, sacrum. Two visits.)

THE *BEST* REASON TO BREAST-FEED

In over 30 years of private practice, the difference between breast-fed and bottle-fed babies has always been perfectly obvious to me. Young mothers who bottle-feed tell me they're frequently in and out of doctors' offices with the baby. Mothers of breast-fed babies say their babies are happy, vibrant and rarely sick.

Bottle-fed babies often develop disorders and infirmities in their first few years, lowering their health, vitality and productivity and incurring medical costs and risk associated with treatment. That's quite an incentive to breast-feed. But there are far greater incentives, and I've seen them in my own children and in my practice: look into the eyes of a bottle-feeding baby and you'll see a lackluster stare. Then study a baby that's breast- feeding and you'll see pure ecstasy. Clearly, breast-feeding meets more than nutritional needs.

An adult analogy would, perhaps, be between a store-bought apple "fresh" out of long-term storage in a warehouse and a just-picked apple from a healthy mountain tree. The store apple brings only calories to the palate, while the mountain apple dazzles it; the store apple disappoints, the mountain apple brings joy!

Dr. Robert Mendohlson writes in his book *The Medical Heretic*, "There are two things that, if used by all mothers, would ruin pediatric practices.... One is breast-feeding ... (t)he other is Grandma." If you breast-feed and listen to grandma's sage advice instead of making unnecessary trips to the pediatrician, you'll have a healthy, happy, robust child.

CHAPTER 9

MEDICINE ALWAYS RESISTS CHANGE

WHY DIDN'T MY DOCTOR
RECOMMEND A CHIROPRACTOR?

I hear that question often and never know how to answer
it succinctly in believable phrases that my listener can
accept. If I try to be brief, what I say seems incredible; if I
go for the long-winded answer, the listener grows bored.

I take little solace in the fact that other chiropractors have
similar problems answering this question. In the preface to
his book *Medicine, Monopolies and Malice: How the
medical establishment tried to destroy chiropractic in the
U.S.* (Avery Publishing, 1996), Dr. Chester A. Wilk
addresses the issues better than I can:

> If chiropractic has all these advantages, why
> doesn't everyone know it? Why are medical
> doctors more likely to refer patients with back pain
> to orthopedists and neurologists, rather than to
> chiropractors? And why is it that most American

hospitals not only have no chiropractic departments but do not have even a single affiliated chiropractor—in spite of the overwhelming evidence of chiropractic's superiority.

These were some of the questions I asked myself over the past 40 years, as I watched my profession struggle. ... When I finally learned the answers, it changed my life. I learned that all of the misconceptions, broken promises, and slammed doors that we chiropractors found ourselves facing every day were no accident, but a product of a calculated campaign by organized medicine that meant to do no less than to destroy our profession.

The answer is so unexpected, so far removed from most people's concept of allopathic medicine that most people find it unbelievable. Before I decided to become a chiropractor, I held the majority opinion that allopathic doctors were god-like authorities on all healthcare-related issues. I grew up thinking that my doctor had my best interests at heart and if questioned would give honest answers that were based in fact. That's how I thought before I became a chiropractor.

What you're about to read does not apply to all medical doctors. It applies to the politics of medicine, in particular the AMA's viperous political stance against chiropractors. Not all MDs endorse the AMA's vicious, unwarranted attack on chiropractic and chiropractors. I have treated four MDs and the spouses of three MDs. During the course of their treatment, each of the doctors expressed surprise that the adjustments were so gentle. Two doctors praised my protocol; one remarked, "Wow; this isn't anything like what they taught us [about chiropractors] in med. school!" That was in 2003.

What follows applies primarily to the organized, political body that is the American Medical Association and to those doctors and affiliated medical organizations that chose/choose to support it without checking the facts for themselves.

Beginning in the late 1950s, the AMA tried very hard to crush chiropractic, going so far as to form a special committee to "first contain and ultimately eliminate" chiropractic. This "anti-quackery" committee adopted ruthless tactics, including lobbying aggressively to prevent government funding for chiropractic colleges. They disseminated anti-chiropractic literature to the media and to Congress. They formulated AMA sanctions forbidding medical doctors from referring patients to chiropractors, from teaching at chiropractic colleges, and even from socializing with "rabid dogs", "killers" and "quacks"—their words for chiropractors, taken from court testimony and reported in Wilk's book.

This anti-chiropractic committee waged war until 1977, when five chiropractors brought suit against the AMA and sixteen other medical organizations for violating monopoly and antitrust statutes (Wilk et al. v. the AMA et al.). Under federal law, it's illegal for any institution to restrict trade in another group. Competition is the heartbeat of a free economy and there are laws in place to protect it.

The discovery phase of the trial ruined my ivory tower image of the medical community and shattered my faith in it. That phase, if memory serves, lasted 24 months or more. The AMA resisted discovery at every opportunity; incriminating documents were conveniently lost and misplaced. (If you've seen the movie "Erin Brockovich", you know what I'm talking about.) Were it not for one brave soul known only as "Sore Throat", many of the vital documents would never have seen the inside of the courtroom. Sore Throat was an AMA insider who leaked information and documents to the plaintiffs' law firm, which I consider an act of bravery that rivals any in a Hollywood movie. Were it not for Sore Throat, I doubt that the chiropractors would have won the suit.

You have never seen a documentary or news report about that David and Goliath trial, though it may have been the biggest healthcare verdict of all time. What, exactly, did chiropractors win? We forced the AMA to issue a public statement saying that its members would no longer be sanctioned for referring patients to chiropractors. That's all.

But my point is not the substance of the lawsuit but the anti-chiropractic attitude and the needless suffering that this prejudice still generates. Asked, "Do you think a chiropractor might help me?" a doctor STILL often answers in the negative. Very often this answer is based upon "trickle-down" misinformation from the AMA's longstanding war on chiropractic.

Although this perspective is gradually changing, there is still a lot of anti-chiropractic prejudice out there. Given the hectic workload of most doctors, one can understand why they might take the easy way out and accept the party line on chiropractic rather than investigate the issue (or the AMA's long history of bigotry) themselves.

Nonetheless, I honestly can't imagine that most doctors would knowingly endorse the AMA's prejudicial and repressive actions against chiropractic. Wouldn't statements such as the one quoted below, from the AMA's Committee on Quackery, alert most ethical doctors to the organization's heavy-handed prejudice? In *Medicine, Monopolies and Malice* (page 45) Dr. Wilk, one of the plaintiffs in the lawsuit, writes:

> The secret internal documents and memos [released by Sore Throat]... shed light on a master plan. They revealed that the AMA had organized and funded a special committee and, according to the book, called it the Committee on Quackery. Actually, the AMA Board of Trustees had first considered calling it the Committee on Chiropractic, but then they decided that this would

dignify our profession. ... [T]his way their efforts could have a more benevolent sound—as though they were cleaning out the quacks within medicine. In reality, the AMA was deeply concerned about competition.

I came to a quote from a memorandum sent from the Committee on Quackery to the AMA Board of Trustees. This document began:

"Since the AMA Board of Trustees' decision, at its meeting on November 2-3, 1963, to establish a Committee on Quackery, your Committee has considered its prime mission to be, first, the containment of chiropractic and, ultimately, the elimination of chiropractic.

"Your Committee believes it is well along in its mission and is, at the same time, moving toward the ultimate goal. This, then, might be considered a progress report on developments in the past seven years. The Committee has not previously submitted such a report because it believes that to make public some of its activities would have been and continues to be unwise. Thus, this report is intended only for the information of the Board of Trustees."

A cold chill of shock went through me. Here was a widely respected professional organization, one of the most powerful lobbying groups in the nation, actively working to eliminate me and my profession!

If you really want to know why your doctor didn't recommend a chiropractor, I suggest that you read Dr. Wilk's book. Prepare to be shocked. In addition to the sanctions listed above, it documents the following AMA activities undertaken to crush chiropractic: Boycott the Kentuckiana Childrens' Center because it used chiropractors and medical doctors together; make it "unethical to refer patients to a chiropractor for any reason whatsoever"; sponsor "research" intended to discredit chiropractic's effectiveness; withhold research proving chiropractic's effectiveness; lobby against chiropractic funding for research and student loans; make every effort to see that Medicare does not cover chiropractic; do everything within its power to keep the U.S. Office of Education from accrediting chiropractic colleges; encourage separation of the two national chiropractic associations (divide and conquer); encourage state medical associations to fight pro-chiropractic legislation;

publicly discredit chiropractic at every opportunity; print anti-chiropractic books, air TV spots, write editorials, etc.; print anti-chiropractic pamphlets and give a copy to every member of Congress; pressure other medical associations to adopt an anti-chiropractic position; oppose chiropractic inroads to health insurance, workers' compensation, labor unions, and hospitals; contain and stifle chiropractic schools.

Containment of chiropractic schools was basic to the AMA plan. Wilk quotes the AMA committee: "Any successful policy of 'containment' of chiropractic, must necessarily be directed at the schools. To the extent that these financial problems continue or multiply, and to the extent that the schools are unsuccessful in their recruiting programs, the chiropractic menace of the future will be reduced and possibly eliminated."

You may think that because that all happened in the 60s and 70s it is part of the past. Or you may think the lawsuit changed the AMA's anti-chiropractic position. I, too, expected the AMA to do a turnaround. Judge Susan Getzendanner ordered the AMA to print publicly that it would no longer punish doctors for referring a patient to a chiropractor. When the statement finally appeared, the word "chiropractor" was nowhere in it! Instead, it referred to us as "limited practitioners" because using the term "chiropractic" would have given us recognition the AMA still considered undeserved. The AMA retained its anti-chiropractic position long after the ink dried on the court order, and it would be naïve to think that real change has been achieved.

Some things are slowly changing, however. Despite the crushing opposition from such a powerful enemy, chiropractic care has continued to slowly gain popularity and support. One can only wonder how much faster our profession would have grown in a less hostile environment.

Today, some chiropractors and doctors do work together. Chiropractors are making inroads into some hospitals. In a few seminars, medical doctors actually lecture with or participate in discussions with chiropractors.

But although the climate is slowly changing, the prejudice is still with us—it has simply gone underground. The AMA no longer punishes doctors for referring to a chiropractor, but we are hardly up to our ears in referrals. In thirty years of practice, I have referred 326 cases to medical doctors. These cases involved problems that were better off being treated by an allopath. It's my legal and ethical duty to refer out any such case. I have had two patients that were direct referrals from medical doctors, one in May 1979, the other on July 13, 2007. I've asked three of my colleagues if they've had referrals from doctors. Two said no, one had had five such referrals over 22 years. Considering how effective chiropractic is for structural pain and how common such pain is, one would expect many more chiropractic referrals from doctors … if only no such prejudice existed.

During the Wilk suit, AMA-sponsored research into chiropractic's effectiveness was entered into evidence. We can assume that the AMA commissioned it in order to gain evidence to discredit chiropractic; instead, it supported the effectiveness of chiropractic. The study was never published by the AMA, but it (and later published reports) showed that for the health problems the AMA researched, chiropractic works twice as fast as most everything else in the medical arsenal. Twice as fast as physical therapy, physiatry, nonsteroidal anti inflammatories, etc. These results came out during the trial. (The AMA shelved their research when it proved to support chiropractic's superior effectiveness for musculoskeletal cases.) To my thinking, if a doctor knows of a better treatment, s/he is not only ethically obligated to disclose this to the patient but would want to do so in the patient's best interests. But prejudice dies hard.

During the antitrust trial, one of the AMA's witnesses disclosed what I believe to be the biggest reason for the prejudice against chiropractic. It has to do with medical school training (or more accurately, the lack of it) in structural complaints. Dr. John McMillan Mennell was testifying. He had authored textbooks and articles and had served as a professor at eight different medical schools. At the time of the trial, he was Professor of Physical Medicine at the University of Connecticut and was one of the few doctors of that era to have publicly visited a chiropractic college. (In Wilk's book, he is quoted as saying that the National College of Chiropractic had the "finest department of anatomy" that he'd ever seen.)

Dr. Mennell testified at the request of the AMA, et al., which apparently wanted his testimony to prove that compared to medical doctors, chiropractors had inadequate training in musculoskeletal manipulation. If the AMA could prove that, it would have a valid excuse to oppose chiropractic. Ironically, Dr. Mennell's testimony helped the plaintiffs. Again, I quote from Wilk's book:

The AMA's attorney asked, "I think you said that medical residents receive four or five hours training in manipulative therapy, is this correct?" Dr. Mennell replied, "I think I said zero hours, didn't I, for the most part?" Apparently finding Dr. Mennell's response hard to believe, the AMA lawyer pressed him further. "What I'm trying to determine is, when you talk about zero hours' training in manipulation, what particular definition of manipulation were you referring to?" Dr. Mennell answered, "I think my testimony was that if you ask a bunch of new residents who come into a hospital for the first time how long they spent in studying the problems of the musculoskeletal system, they would, for the most part, reply, 'zero to about four hours'. I think that was my testimony." The attorney asked, "the musculoskeletal system comprises what portion of the body?" "As a system, about 60 percent of the body."

"Is your testimony ... that the residents to whom you just referred told you they had no training whatsoever relating to problems as to 60 percent of the body?" Dr. Mennell replied, "That is just about right." Once again, the AMA's lawyer seemed to be astonished at Dr. Mennell's testimony. "Is it your testimony that it is your understanding that the entire medical school curriculum is devoted to about 40 percent of the body?" Without hesitation, Dr. Mennell answered, "Yes, sir."

The above quotation clearly reflects part of the problem between chiropractors and medical doctors. We chiropractors spend over 1000 hours studying the musculoskeletal system; in 1977 doctors spent zero to four hours studying it. No wonder they considered what we do to be irrelevant— they got that message in medical school!

So, to sum up, you should not be surprised that your pediatrician didn't refer you to a chiropractor. Perhaps you should be outraged, instead. The data reflecting chiropractic's success with colic are out there, just a click away on the Internet where anyone, including a pediatrician, can read it. So instead of asking me, you might want to ask your pediatrician why s/he didn't tell you about the most effective treatment for colic. I guess I actually do have a short answer to the question: "Please, go ask your doctor!"

YOU AND I ARE MAKING HISTORY

The medical community has always been resistant to and prejudiced against any new thing. As early as 1553 Servetus wrote a book describing pulmonary circulation. The medical experts burned his books and only three survived. Fifty years later, medicine accepted Servetus' views, even though one dissection would have verified them. Leonardo Da Vinci's works on anatomy were seized by medical experts and burned in the public square. Two hundred years later, medicine caught up with his theories.

In Vienna, Ignaz Semmelweiss (1818-1865) spent years trying to prove the connection between maternal death and the fact that doctors rarely washed their hands, even after performing autopsies. The infant death rate hovered near 70 percent and one in five mothers died.

Semmelweiss thought something was hitchhiking from the morgue and infecting the babies and mothers. To test his theory, he had to ask his colleagues to wash their hands.

At first, the medical community ostracized Semmelweiss, but his persistence paid off and doctors started washing their hands. Infant mortality dropped to around 15 percent. Suddenly, doctors were blamed for all the prior deaths, and they retaliated against Semmelweiss by not washing. The death rates went back up. They had Dr. Semmelweiss declared insane and institutionalized— ironically enough, directly across the street from the hospital. He died in his cell at the asylum, and it was 80 years before medicine grudgingly admitted to the presence of germs and their role in "childbirth fever".

Florence Nightingale noticed that hospitals were filthy places where wounded men often slept on sheets soiled and bloodied by the previous occupant. She noted the proliferation of rats, the bloody floors, walls, and, especially, doctor's aprons, and wondered if fewer men would die if only hospitals were clean. She was harassed and ridiculed for her theories. Doctors of that era felt that blood and spatter were a sign of prestige. It took decades of strong-willed persistence and stubborn, selfless sacrifice to get doctors to advance that thinking, to wash their hands and wear clean clothes.

Madame Curie's discovery of x-ray was scorned, and the medical arena scoffed at her work because she was "just a woman". The Palmer School of Chiropractic was the first healthcare institution to buy and use her machines, and chiropractors were taking x-rays (then called "spinographs") long before medicine adopted x-ray technology.

In more recent times, Linus Pauling (1901-1994) was ridiculed and scorned for suggesting that Vitamin C would prevent the common cold and other infections. After several decades, and much money and effort, the medical community was forced to stop laughing at his work. Pauling eventually won the Nobel Prize for his work.

 My point is that medicine resists change, even when it might help patients. It has been so in the past. It is so in the present. It will continue to be so in the future.

One day, decades from now, organized, political medicine will be forced to accept our drugless, natural healthcare paradigm. The neurology proves it. The anatomy proves it. The subluxation-correction methodology is here, and so are the chiropractors who practice it. It will still take many years for the medical power structure to accept as fact that chiropractic care might help humanity.

By using chiropractic as a valid treatment for your baby's colic, you're a part of history in the making. When enough patients respond favorably, the medical community will have no choice but to accept, however grudgingly, that chiropractic care is the only sane, effective treatment for colic and some other problems. They will do that only when public support reaches a critical mass.

I feel that restoring bliss to babies is a great way to start the ball rolling.

In this age of instant information when nearly everyone owns or has access to a computer, TV and cell phone, I continue to be amazed at how surprisingly few people *still* don't know about chiropractic's remarkable benefits.

If I had to sum up everything I know about chiropractic care and colicky babies I would say: chiropractic works better than anything else, with an average 92 percent success rate. Don't just take my word for it; try it. Results speak louder than words.

The next step toward sweet dreams for your baby is yours to take.

ABOUT THE AUTHOR

I graduated from Palmer College of Chiropractic in Davenport Iowa in 1977, the same year I married my wife, Jo, whom I love more every day. We have two grown children, Aaron and Kelly. I have maintained a private practice in Northern California since 1977. My post-graduate and extracurricular training are listed below.

Some people can't enter a room without straightening a crooked picture. I have a similar compulsion, a passion to set subluxated spines right, and when a patient gets well as a result of my care, I feel joy. Often, this is a patient has already been to several doctors, without resolution. I'd be lying if I said that I take no pride in my successes.

I adjusted my first patient in 1976, a child of seven who had had constant nosebleeds for five weeks despite cauterization and blood-thickening drugs. In chiropractic, we're trained to look for causes, instead of symptoms. So, I looked and found an obvious subluxation at the third cervical vertebra—a rare subluxation pattern that produced a rare symptom, nosebleeds. I adjusted the child, the bleeding stopped, permanently, in about thirty seconds. So, since my very first adjustment, I've been deeply aware of the value of chiropractic for children. I still feel a thrill when I think of the wonderful effect that adjustment had on the child, and I get that same thrill today when I adjust people. If I ever lose it, I'll retire and devote myself exclusively to my other interests—archery, fishing, camping and wildlife photography.

PROFESSIONAL TRAINING

Most students of chiropractic study, on average, three primary techniques. As practitioners, they then either blend these techniques or concentrate on just one to the point of specializing in it. I have made it a point to get training in as wide a variety of techniques as possible and to learn from as many masters as possible. In part, I got the broadest training possible simply out of intellectual curiosity. But it also has proven to serve my patients well, for I've found that while a given technique may work well on eight patients out of ten, two won't get relief. If I can switch from approach A to B or C or even D, the more likely I am to be able to treat a broad range of cases successfully. What follows is a condensed list of the graduate and postgraduate courses I've taken. I include it here to provide a glimpse into the breadth and depth of chiropractic training that is available.

<u>1974-77 Palmer College of Chiropractic (PCC), Davenport, Iowa</u>. The training to obtain a DC degree is usually a four-year curriculum. I studied at an accelerated pace, year-round for 36 months. The instruction I received was typical for any of the good chiropractic colleges of that time and included gross anatomy, dissection, spinal anatomy, physiology, organic chemistry, biochemistry, angiology, splanchnology, histology, neurology (CNS and Peripheral NS), physical diagnosis, parasitology and communicability, basic laboratory procedures, chiropractic exams, x-ray physics, darkroom techniques, x-ray clinical (patient positioning and safety), radiology (reading x-rays for pathology, etc.,) x-ray analysis, physical therapy, emergency procedures (CPR, first aid), chiropractic philosophy, ethics and jurisprudence. I also learned the Palmer Technique of chiropractic adjusting which included courses in Upper Cervical, Diversified and Gonstead techniques.

During my years at Palmer, I also attended a wide range of extracurricular seminars. These ranged in length from one to sixteen days and from 8 to 96 hours. They were taught by professionals from the United States, South America, Australia and Europe. Several of the seminars included techniques relevant to treating babies, among them: the Gillet Motion Palpation Seminar (digital palpation of articular structures during passive normal motion, including baby techniques); Toftness Non-Force Technique (an extremely light force technique using Toftness' patented TRD and stylus); Basic Sacro Occipital Technique and Advanced SOT. SOT is a physical chiropractic analysis system that includes assessment and technique for babies.

Other seminars I attended while at Palmer included: Erhardt Disc Adjustment, Ehmann Non-Force Technique (a spin-off from Van Rumpt's work, with an emphasis on viscerosomatic reflexes of a dietary nature); Terminal Point Drop; Receptor-Tonus (the first digital goading treatment method, highly effective for chronic and centralized pain); Beginning Applied Kinesiology and Advanced Applied Kinesiology (a system of physical analysis—the training includes baby technique, chronic and difficult cases, gravity stress analysis, special challenges, soft tissue challenges and cranial adjusting); Extremity Challenges and Adjusting. I was certified as an Advanced AK practitioner in 1977. I took the Erhardt Postgraduate Radiological Seminars, Motion Palpation Institute Seminar, Receptor-Tonus, and several 12-hour seminars in appendicular and costosternal adjusting.

Postgraduate Training. After beginning my practice, I have kept up my habit of attending seminars that present techniques and theories I wish to explore. I attend annual seminars in technique that are *required* for a chiropractor's license to be renewed. I attended the Ninth Annual Interdisciplinary Conference on the Spine; PCRF Seminars in activator, nutrition, and gait analysis arch measurements (for fitting Foot Levelers); Erhardt Postgraduate Radiological Seminars, Activator Methods; complete extremity adjusting technique; introduction to Cox-Leander distraction technique for diagnosing and treating lumbar disc herniation; Interpreting Magnetic Resonance Imaging with special attention to the cord and spinal canal and knowing when to refer cases to medical specialists; Kontz Adjusting Seminar (terminal point drop technique); three years' attendance at "The Class", a seminar focusing on full spine and extremity techniques and clinical procedures, including on-site injury treatment for musculoskeletal conditions); Barge Chiropractic Seminars on

133

Scoliosis (including impact of the Heuter-Volkmann Phenomenon on pre-adolescent subluxation, disc-block theory, infragenic and supragenic subluxation patterns, x-ray analysis, heel lift theory and application).

Baby Technique. A few additional observations on the training listed above that I've found of particular value with respect to my work with babies:

- The obstetrics/gynecology class that I took while at Palmer was taught by Maxine McMullen, DC. She was a midwife in Australia before she became a Palmer chiropractor and an excellent chiropractic instructor. Her warm style and her fervent pro-baby attitude motivated me to treat babies.
- Sacro Occipital Technique (SOT) is a physical chiropractic analysis system that includes management for adjusting babies. I was certified as an Advanced SOT practitioner in 1977.
- In contrast to SOT cranial, Applied Kinesology (AK) cranial utilizes active rather than passive assessment of the cranial sutures. I prefer AK for my cranial work with both adults and infants. I was certified as an Advanced AK practitioner in 1977.
- In 1980, '84 and '85, I attended seminars given by Dr. Fuhr and Dr. Lee, who focused on the percussion instrument known as an Activator. A six-inch, spring-loaded, plunger-like device, it has a soft tip that can deliver an adjustable amount of pressure with relative precision. Dr. Fuhr's seminars included training in his meticulous pre-adjustment assessment protocol. This protocol is to establish the proper segmental contact point, line of correction, and thrust setting, as well as knowing where and when to adjust, and more importantly, when *not* to adjust. In teaching baby technique, Dr. Fuhr emphasizes the use of the "Baby Tip" on the instrument, a soft silicone sleeve that ensures an especially gentle adjustment.

GLOSSARY OF TERMS

ACUTE—Any injury or condition that has existed in the body only for a short time is said to be acute. For insurance purposes, this means fewer than 90 days. "Acute" is not a measure of severity; a problem can be both minor and acute... as in "acute skin rash".

ADJUSTMENT—This term includes the whole chiropractic procedure: the evaluation and preparation before the chiropractic thrust, the thrust and the post-check. Chiropractic has used this term since its earliest days to distinguish what we do from every other thing in healthcare. It is not a "manipulation", although current medical terminology is trying to overpower chiropractic's uniqueness by using terms like "Spinal Manipulative Therapy", "complementary alternative medicine", and other philosophically erosive phrases. The chiropractic term "adjustment" was adopted with scrupulous attention to terminology. It is distinctly opposed to "manipulations", which were used by osteopathy, naturopathy and homeopathy. "Manipulation" is a term used to describe a therapeutic mobilization of soft tissue, blood vessels, skin and fat in order to reverse a disease process. The adjustment is performed upon subluxated vertebrae, with the express purpose of correcting nerve interference and not to achieve any specific therapeutic effect or to reverse or control anything. Adjustments are performed upon specific contact points—e.g., the transverse process, the spinous process, the mammillary process or other prominent vertebral leverage points. Adjustments are also known as SLHVLA thrusts, which stands for "Short Lever, High Velocity, Low Amplitude" thrust vectors, which are intended to correct specific subluxations.

ADVERSE DRUG REACTION—Also known as an "adverse drug event", this is a reaction to a drug that is not desired. An ADR can be mild or fatal, self-limiting or permanent. Most are self-limiting and minor. Every drug can cause such a reaction.

ALLOPATHY—This is the term for conventional Western medicine, currently the largest branch of the healing arts. This term comes from two root words, "allo", meaning reverse, and "pathy", meaning symptom or disease process. Allopathy is at its finest when treating patients with life-threatening injuries and major disease processes, and those needing surgical procedures.

ARTICULATION—This is a fancy word for a joint. Articular surfaces in a joint are those surfaces that facilitate movement of that joint.

APPLIED KINESIOLOGY—This field of chiropractic analysis works with the body's energy systems. It relies heavily upon specific manual muscle testing to detect imbalances in the body. Treatment involves reflex points on the body, including neurolymphatic and neurovascular reflexes, chiropractic adjustment, meridian therapy and other natural methods to balance muscle strength. With the immediate feedback available, an AK chiropractor can and often does bring about dramatic and swift improvements; many times after other methods have failed.

ATLAS—The uppermost vertebra, named after Atlas, the mythological god who held up the world. So named, because of its tiny size and massive job of holding up the head. This extreme task subjects Atlas to unique subluxation insult patterns, especially in babies. The atlas provides most of the flexion/extension for the head (i.e., nodding).

AXIS—The second highest vertebra, providing much of the rotation in the cervical spine.

BACK—Most people use this term to describe the low back, as opposed to the thoracic spine or the cervical spine. However, "back" generally means anything from T 1, the highest of the vertebrae, to the coccyx or lowest vertebrae.

CARTILAGE—Connective issue that fits between two bones in order to cushion them from load bearing shock. Most joints have cartilage pads in them.

CERVICAL— Referring to the topmost vertebrae, those in the neck. The first seven vertebrae (C 1 to C 7) below the skull are the "cervicals".

CEREBROSPINAL FLUID—This bathes and protects the brain and spinal cord. It circulates from the brain down to the lower tip of the cord and back up again. Specialized organs manufacture CSF from the blood stream. There are no white blood cells in the CSF. This is why a spinal infection is so dangerous. CSF carries sugar and oxygen to the nerve system and is the only source of nutrition for the brain and cord. Your CSF is constantly being produced and simultaneously reabsorbed, so that your precise level of CSF is maintained. Too low or too high a level of CSF can cause serious physical problems.

CHIROPRACTIC (Cairo-prak-tik)—This term comes from two Greek roots, Cheir (hand) and Praktos (practice, or to do). So the term means, quite simply, done by hand. This noun has no plural form. We don't say "chiropractics", "chiropractory" or "chiropractic medicine". The theory behind chiropractic is that spinal dysfunction predisposes the body to suboptimal homeostatic conditions. Left in place for enough time, these dysfunctions or "subluxations" pose a significant vector of suboptimal functioning, which can result in illness. Chiropractic care centers on manual correction of subluxations, as well as on the hygienic measures available to all physicians—diet, exercise, mental, emotional and spiritual health, etc. Chiropractic is not a treatment for disease, it does not attempt to reverse symptoms or otherwise manipulate the body's internal regulatory systems. Its specific intent is to remove barriers to optimal health ... without the use of drugs or surgery.

CHIROPRACTIC DOCTOR—The DC (Doctor of Chiropractic) is a practitioner of chiropractic. The chiropractic doctor practices drugless, natural healthcare. At the very root of the practice is the attention to spinal health, including but not limited to spinal adjustments.

CHRONIC—Any injury or condition that has existed in the body for a long period of time is said to be "chronic". For insurance purposes, this is over 90 days in duration. "Chronic" is <u>not</u> a measure of severity but of duration.

CONNECTIVE TISSUE—This is the substance that "connects" many of the elements in your body. For example, epimyseum is a connective tissue. It surrounds muscle groups and blends into the ending tendon for the muscle, rather like Saran Wrap. CT performs several important functions; it connects, it binds, wraps and even insulates certain structures. It is also very richly endowed with pain sensors in order to give the brain feedback when injury or insult occurs. Without this feedback, further injury to a structure would certainly occur.

CORTEX—The outer layer of some organs and structures is called the cortex. You have a cerebral cortex, which is the outer layer of the brain. Similarly, the adrenal glands have a cortex, the source of cortico-steroids. The cortex of the bones is the hard, dense outer part. Think of the cortex as the outer layer of something—the peel of an orange, for example.

DISC—These are unique structures deep inside the spine. In between two vertebrae, the disc provides for mobility. Discs are made up of connective tissue. In each disc's center is a gelatin-like substance called the nucleus pulposis. It provides a pivot point around which the vertebrae are able to move in a limited fashion. Each pair of vertebrae encloses a disc, except in the highest part of the neck, where the skull, Atlas and Axis have no discs in the top articulations.

HOMEOPATHY—This healthcare system derives its philosophy from its root words: "Homeo", meaning same, and "pathy", meaning symptom or illness. It is a system of treating disease that is based upon the premise that "like cures like"—a teeny bit of the same thing that made you sick can make you well. Remedies in homeopathy are extremely diluted elixirs aimed only at triggering your body's inherent curative mechanisms.

HOMEOSTASIS—The roots of this term are homeo, meaning "same", and stasis, meaning "to stay". In science, this word reflects the basic concept of life. All living organisms continually strive for optimum survival parameters. For example, when you're cold, you shiver. Muscle contractions make heat. Heat warms your body. Soon you reach optimum temperature. Shivering stops. When you're hot, you sweat. This cools your body. When optimum has been reached, sweating stops. These and countless other processes all serve to maintain your homeostasis or biological comfort zone. Subluxations are one form of threat to homeostasis.

HEUTER-VOLKMAN PHENOMENON—When bone is subjected to mechanical/gravitational stress, the bone elicits an electrical charge. This causes new bone cells to be laid down in reaction to the stresses. The development of scoliosis can be explained biomechanically on the basis of the Heuter-Volkmann phenomenon, which states that pressure on epiphysis (the growth plate on a bone) retards the rate of growth and that tension increases the rate of growth. Hence, the leading edge of the deformity grows more rapidly than the trailing edge, increasing the rate of progression. The H-V effect can cause huge disturbances in bone growth. In children, when a subluxated vertebra 'tilts', its lower side takes more weight and grows more slowly while the high side bears less weight and grows normally, eventually causing the spine above that vertebra to curve.

IDIOPATHIC—The term for a disease or condition of unknown origin.
INTERVERTEBRAL—This refers to all structures that lie between two vertebrae, among them the intervertebral discs, the spinal nerve root pairs and other structures as well.

139

INTERVERTEBRAL FORAMEN (IVF)—This is the opening through which the spinal nerve exits the spinal column to the target organs. The IVF is composed of a notch in the upper vertebrae, a notch in the lower vertebrae, and the disc. Since either vertebra can subluxate, and therefore compromise the IVF, the structure of the IVF creates a unique environment for nerve root dysfunction. Inside the IVF are structures of vast importance: the artery and vein, the spinal nerve root, lymphatic vessels and the dural sleeve. Chiropractic care places great emphasis upon the IVF's health and well being.

KINESIOLOGY—The study of the body as it moves, kinesiology is common domain to trainers, therapists, coaches and anyone else in a variety of fields. It is to be distinguished from "applied kinesiology", in which chiropractors apply chiropractic principles to the science of kinesiology in order to get people well faster.

LIGAMENT—The inelastic connective tissue that spans a joint, starting at one bone and ending at another bone. The purpose of a ligament is to prevent joint motion that is excessive or damaging to the joint. No muscles are attached to a ligament. Another function of ligaments is to preserve architectural integrity, such as in the arches of the foot. Think of ligaments as chains that tether one bone to another.

LUMBAR—The lumbar spine lies between the thoracic spine and the sacrum. Normally consisting of five moveable vertebrae (L 1 to L5), some lumbar spines have six segments, while others contain only four vertebrae. While these variations are considered "normal anatomical variants", they can predispose one to protracted and frequent back pain.
LYMPH—This thin, watery fluid, produced by the lymph glands, travels throughout the body via tiny vein-like tubes. Lymph is vital to the musculoskeletal system's well being and is also a key component in the body's ability to fend off infections.

LYMPHATICS—This term refers to the lymph and its circulatory system. The lymphatic system depends upon very slight pressure gradients to achieve its circulation. These pressure gradients come from gravity, breathing and muscular activity.

MUSCLE—This elastic tissue provides motion for the body. Muscles come in three forms: "skeletal", which cause joints to move, "smooth", which cause digestion and elimination to occur, and "cardiac", which is a mixture of the first two types.

NEUROLYMPHATIC—In Applied Kinesiology we use "neurolymphatic" points, which are hypothesized to bolster lymphatic drainage of certain muscles and organs. Improved lymphatic circulation is thought to result in improved health.

NEUROVASCULAR—In Applied Kinesiology we use "neurovascular" reflex points, which are hypothesized to enhance micro-circulation in muscles and organs. As with neurolymphatic points, there's no current technology to prove the efficacy of these points, but they seem to work.

OSTEOPATHY—The healthcare discipline that fits in between chiropractic and allopathic medicine, osteopathy is a good method of medical healthcare even though its critics claim that it's "neither fish nor fowl". Osteopathic doctors do good things for their patients and are interested in the whole body, lifestyle, etc.

SCOLIOSIS—An abnormal curvature of the spine that can be due to disease processes such as polio or can be idiopathic. Generally, the earlier a person acquires scoliosis, the more severe it can be. (See Heuter-Volkman, above.)

SELF-LIMITING—Any infirmity, ailment or illness that is normally corrected by the body is a self-limiting condition ... one that will get better whether or not you seek medical attention. The common cold is one example of the 80 percent of all medically diagnosed conditions that are self-limiting.

SPINE—The human spine is composed of 24 moveable bones, called vertebrae, and 8 fused bones in the pelvis, called the sacrum (four) and the coccyx (4). Of the body's 601 muscles, 358 attach to the spine. Each of the 24 moveable vertebrae moves a slight amount, giving a wide range of flexibility and motion. In fact, the human spine performs a wider range of movements than the spine of any other species.

STRESS—Any physical, chemical or psychological threat can produce stress. Stress can be good or bad. Good stress, or "eustress", can result from exercise, laughter, seeing a scary movie or taking a roller coaster ride. Eustress causes our bodies and minds to develop, learn and grow. Bad stress, or "dystress", can be result from fear or other negative emotion, repetitive stress to the joints, alcohol or drug addiction, etc. Dystress causes us harm.

STRESSOR—Any variable that creates stimulus is a stressor. If you are studying rats and put one in a pool of water, that's a stressor. If you heat the water, that's a second stressor. When stressors are removed, an organism returns to homeostasis. Spinal subluxation is a significant stressor in the human health equation. Removing this stressor will often allow the body to get well again.

TENDON—Ropy tissue that connects a muscle to a bone and makes motion possible. When the tendon moves, the joint moves. When a muscle contracts, a joint will move thanks to the tendon.

THORACIC—The thorax consists of the ribs, thoracic vertebrae, the sternum, the heart and lungs. However, when chiropractors speak of "thoracics", we are referring to the vertebrae in that region, T1 – T12.

THRUST—Chiropractors often use this term interchangeably with "adjustment". Technically, the thrust is the physical attempt to correct a subluxation, while an "adjustment" is the entire process that results in subluxation correction. Thrusts come in several types—manual, where the doctor uses his/her hands; mechanical, where the DC uses an instrument; and "light force", which involves very subtle forces, such as the SOT blocks. The most widely used is the "Short Lever, High Velocity, Low Amplitude" dynamic thrust. This is the classic "audible" adjustment that has been the exclusive domain of chiropractic for the past hundred years. Unfortunately, some medical doctors and even physical therapists now attempt to perform SLHVLA thrusts without having adequate chiropractic training. This is doubtlessly due to the public's keen interest in chiropractic's effectiveness. Imitation may be the sincerest form of flattery, but *this* type is not; it puts the public at undue risk and it deceives the 'customer'.

VERTEBRA—An individual spinal bone of irregular shape, a vertebra has several functions. It protects the spinal cord, it allows for upright posture and it provides motion via its interlocking system of joints. The vertebrae also produce blood cells, and the spine is a major blood cell producer in adults.

www.ingramcontent.com/pod-product-compliance
Lightning Source LLC
Chambersburg PA
CBHW071002040426
42443CB00007B/627